# Aging Medicine

Robert Pignolo, MD, PhD; Mary Ann Forciea, MD;
Jerry C. Johnson, MD, Series Editors



For other titles published in this series, go to
www.springer.com/series/7622

# Life-Span Extension

## Single-Cell Organisms to Man


Edited by

Christian Sell, PhD
Department of Pathology and Laboratory Medicine
Drexel University College of Medicine, Philadelphia, PA, USA

Antonello Lorenzini, PhD
Department of Pathology, and Laboratory Medicine
Drexel University College of Medicine, Philadelphia, PA, USA

Holly M. Brown-Borg, PhD
Department of Pharmacology, Physiology and Therapeutics
School of Medicine and Health Sciences, University of North Dakota
Grand Forks, ND, USA


Humana Press

*Editors*
Christian Sell
Department of Pathology
and Laboratory Medicine
Drexel University
College of Medicine
Philadelphia, PA
USA

Antonello Lorenzini
Department of Pathology
and Laboratory Medicine
Drexel University
College of Medicine
Philadelphia, PA
USA

Holly M. Brown-Borg
Department of Pharmacology,
Physiology and Therapeutics
School of Medicine and Health Sciences
University of North Dakota
Grand Forks, ND
USA

ISBN: 978-1-60327-506-4 e-ISBN: 978-1-60327-507-1
DOI 10.1007/978-1-60327-507-1
Springer Dordrecht Heidelberg London New York

Library of Congress Control Number: 2009922206



*Cover illustration:* Christian Sell, PhD

Printed on acid-free paper

Springer is part of Springer Science+Business Media (www.springer.com)

# Preface

This volume contains viewpoints of investigators studying the aging process in species ranging from yeast to man. The effort to compile these viewpoints has been driven by recent, remarkable discoveries about the underlying mechanisms important to aging. Single mutations that extend life span have been identified in yeast, worms, flies, and mice. Studies in humans have identified potentially important markers for successful aging. The genes and pathways identified in these studies involve a surprisingly small set of conserved functions, most of which have been the focus of aging research for some time. For example, recent genome-wide analyses of genes involved in life-span extension that are common to yeast and *Caenorhabditis elegans* identified a regulator of protein synthesis, the mTOR pathway, which leads to transcriptional control as a common longevity pathway in these two organisms. In mammals, this pathway intersects with neuroendocrine pathways and with the insulin/insulin-like growth factor (IGF) pathways, which have been identified as major modulators of life span and aging in both invertebrates and mice. Interestingly, both these pathways interact with stress responses to alter activity in response to environmental conditions. Thus, the emerging technologies and wide variety of systems that are now used to study aging and the mechanisms of aging provide enormous opportunities for the identification of common pathways that modulate longevity. It is these common pathways that are the focus of this volume.

Christian Sell — Philadelphia, PA
Antonello Lorenzini — Philadelphia, PA
Holly M. Brown-Borg — Grand Forks, ND

# Contents

# Contributors

**Robert Arking**
Department of Biological Sciences and Institute of Gerontology, Wayne State University, Detroit, MI, USA

**Marta Artal-Sanz**
Institute of Molecular Biology and Biotechnology, Foundation for Research and Technology, Heraklion, Crete, Greece

**Elena Bellavista**
Department of Experimental Pathology, University of Bologna, Bologna, Italy
C.I.G.-Interdepartmental Centre "L. Galvani," University of Bologna, Bologna, Italy

**Kurt E. Borg**
School of Medicine and Health Sciences, University of North Dakota, Grand Forks, ND, USA

**Éric Le Bourg**
Université Paul-Sabatier Centre de Recherche sur la Cognition Animale, Toulouse, France

**Holly M. Brown-Borg**
School of Medicine and Health Sciences, University of North Dakota, Grand Forks, ND, USA

**Rochelle Buffenstein**
The Sam and Ann Barshop Institute for Longevity and Aging Studies and Department of Physiology, University of Texas Health Science Center at San Antonio, San Antonio, TX, USA

**Miriam Capri**
Department of Experimental Pathology, University of Bologna, Bologna, Italy
C.I.G.-Interdepartmental Centre "L. Galvani," University of Bologna, Bologna, Italy

**Laura Celani**
Department of Experimental Pathology, University of Bologna, Bologna, Italy
C.I.G.-Interdepartmental Centre "L. Galvani," University of Bologna, Bologna, Italy

**Alessandro Cellerino**
Fritz-Lipmann Institute for Age Research, Beutenbergstr.11, Jena, Germany.

**Elisa Cevenini**
Department of Experimental Pathology, University of Bologna, Bologna, Italy
C.I.G.-Interdepartmental Centre "L. Galvani," University of Bologna, Bologna, Italy

**Sean P. Curran**
Department of Molecular Biology, Massachusetts General Hospital, and Department of Genetics, Harvard Medical School, Boston, MA, USA

**Yael H. Edrey**
The Sam and Ann Barshop Institute for Longevity and Aging Studies and the Department of Physiology, University of Texas Health Science Center at San Antonio, San Antonio, TX, USA

**Claudio Franceschi**
Department of Experimental Pathology, University of Bologna, Bologna, Italy
C.I.G.-Interdepartmental Centre "L. Galvani," University of Bologna, Bologna, Italy

**Catia Lanzarini**
Department of Experimental Pathology, University of Bologna, Bologna, Italy
C.I.G.-Interdepartmental Centre "L. Galvani," University of Bologna, Bologna, Italy

**Francesco Lescai**
Department of Experimental Pathology, University of Bologna, Bologna, Italy
C.I.G.-Interdepartmental Centre "L. Galvani," University of Bologna, Bologna, Italy

**Valter D. Longo**
Andrus Gerontology Center and Department of Biological Sciences, University of Southern California, Los Angeles, CA, USA

**Stella Lukas**
Department of Experimental Pathology, University of Bologna, Bologna, Italy
C.I.G.-Interdepartmental Centre "L. Galvani," University of Bologna, Bologna, Italy

**Edward J. Masoro**
The Sam and Ann Barshop Institute for Longevity and Aging Studies, University of Texas Health Science Center, San Antonio, TX, USA

**Michelle E. Matzko**
Center for Developmental and Health Genetics, The Pennsylvania State University, University Park, PA, USA

**Roger J. McCarter**
Center for Developmental and Health Genetics, The Pennsylvania State University, University Park, PA, USA

**Daniela Monti**
Department of Experimental Pathology and Oncology, University of Florence, Florence, Italy

**Sharlene G. Rakoczy**
School of Medicine and Health Sciences, University of North Dakota, Grand Forks, ND, USA

**Stefano Salvioli**
Department of Experimental Pathology, University of Bologna, Bologna, Italy
C.I.G.-Interdepartmental Centre "L. Galvani," University of Bologna, Bologna, Italy

**Christian Sell**
Department of Pathology and Laboratory Medicine, Drexel University College of Medicine, Philadelphia, PA, USA

**Federica Sevini**
Department of Experimental Pathology, University of Bologna, Bologna, Italy
C.I.G.-Interdepartmental Centre "L. Galvani," University of Bologna, Bologna, Italy

**Sunita Sharma**
School of Medicine and Health Sciences, University of North Dakota, Grand Forks, ND, USA

**Nektarios Tavernarakis**
Institute of Molecular Biology and Biotechnology, Foundation for Research and Technology, Heraklion, Crete, Greece

**Paolo Tieri**
Department of Experimental Pathology, University of Bologna, Bologna, Italy
C.I.G.-Interdepartmental Centre "L. Galvani," University of Bologna, Bologna, Italy

# Introduction

**Christian Sell**

**Keywords** Aging • life span • evolution • nutrient • stress

**Abbreviations** DMBA: Dimethylbenzanthracene; IGF: Insulin-like growth factor mTOR: Mammalian target of rapamycin

## 1 Introduction

The chapters presented in this book deal with a variety of species and approaches to research into the basic mechanisms of aging. Placing such a broad collection into perspective can be difficult for those who are new to the area. This introduction provides background and perspective on the aging process. First, two terms that are widely used in aging research, aging and life span, are discussed because the usage and implications of these two terms are important to understanding research related to aging. Next, a conceptual framework is discussed that may provide a useful approach to organizing the information presented in the various chapters regarding multiple influences on longevity.

## 2 Aging vs. Life Span

In considering the impact of gene mutations on aging and life span, it is important to clarify the difference between these two terms. Considerable confusion exists in the general public and, to some degree, in the scientific community regarding the precise usage of the terms aging and life span *(1)*. A potentially useful distinction may be made if one considers that aging occurs within a given population. The term aging refers to the constellation of changes that occurs during the later stages of the life span of any species. Although broad, one potentially useful description of the phenotypic effects of these changes is that an aging organism shows a reduced capacity to maintain homeostasis. This description encompasses most if not all of the characteristics associated with aging such as reduced functional capacity, increased vulnerability to multiple diseases, and a reduction in the ability to respond to stress or injury. Thus, gene mutations or environmental factors such as caloric restriction that have been found to delay the aging process provide improvements in a specific set of cellular or physiologic parameters late in life relative to control populations.

The term life span can be used in several contexts. It can refer either to the life span of a given population under study or to the species life span. Changes in the rate of aging can affect the life span of the study population but may not influence species life span. Species life span remains fixed within a certain limit, although what this limit may be is a matter of some debate *(2, 3)*. For example, caloric restriction will increase the life span of a given population but has not been shown to affect the life span of the species. Thus, there are two key questions concerning life span: *(1)* What mechanisms influence population life span and *(2)* what mechanisms determine the life-span characteristic of a species. These are two different questions. Most of the chapters in this volume deal with population life span. Only those that deal with the comparative biology of aging address the issue of differences between species.

A discussion of aging and its manifestations is provided by Dr. Arking in his chapter, "Overview of the Genetic Architecture of Aging." Dr. Arking provides a detailed analysis of differing life-span curves, indicating that multiple mechanisms underlie changes in life span. It seems to be the complex relationship between environmental influences and the response of the organism to these influences that culminate in the life-span characteristic of a given population. Given the complexity of interactions that dictate life span, it is surprising that common mechanisms would be apparent between divergent species. Recent evidence demonstrates commonalities in the functional pathways (at the level of both the cell and the organism) that respond to environmental influences that are ultimately responsible for life-span changes. Both targeted interventions, such as caloric restriction and gene manipulation, have identified what appear to be general pathways with the ability to modulate life span.

When discussing pathways that modulate aging and life span, one framework that might be useful for the layperson would be to group these pathways into general categories based on the timing of their response to environmental changes. The first category would be rapidly responding pathways. These pathways are involved in the response of the organism to acute stress (such as oxidation), toxicity, and damage; the second category of pathways would be moderately responding pathways, such as those that react more slowly to changes in environmental factors such as nutrient availability; the third category would be slowly responding pathways. This third category includes pathways critical for genomic integrity and other basic functions that would not be expected to undergo rapid alterations. Pathways in all three categories are essential for the organism and may respond to evolutionary pressures to produce a given phenotype.

Examples of rapidly responding pathways are discussed by Dr. Le Bourg. Multiple forms of mild stress such as hypergravity can increase life span in

*Drosophila melanogaster*. Although the mechanisms are not well understood, they include heat shock factors such as hsp70. The response to mild stress is rapid, yet it serves to produce an extension in life span that is a secondary outcome of the primary response.

One could also include the oxygen scavenging enzymes central to free radical theories of aging [see Muller et al. *(4)* for review] and the phase 1 detoxification enzymes in the first category of pathways. The phase 1 enzymes include the heme-containing cytochrome P450 family of enzymes, a large family of enzymes involved in the removal of hydrophobic chemicals from the organism as well as several biosynthetic pathways including cholesterol and bile acid synthesis *(5)*. The expression of the P450 enzymes is affected by exposure to toxins, and altered expression of a subset of the cytochrome P450 enzymes has been described in long-lived, growth hormone-deficient mouse strains *(6)*. It must be borne in mind, however, that the cytochrome P450 enzymes act not only to remove xenobiotics but also to activate carcinogens such as DMBA, creating reactive intermediates. Increased production of such reactive intermediates may increase cancer incidence and contribute to tissue damage. Thus the involvement of this system in modulating life span is likely to be complex [see Nebert and Dalton *(5)* for a discussion of this area].

The second category of pathways includes the neuroendocrine axis (growth hormone, IGF) and the mTOR pathway. These pathways have been the subject of considerable interest in the aging community in recent years. The chapters contributed by Drs. Brown-Borg et al., Matzko et al., and Longo consider this second category of pathways. Acting through mechanisms that are not yet completely clear, it seems that nutrient intake interacts with an organism's developmental program to accelerate or delay development, depending on the relative abundance of food. The highly conserved natures of the pathways that respond to changes in nutrient status reflect the basic need of all organisms for energy input.

The chapter by Dr. Tavernarakis and colleague explores the conserved nature in nematodes of the relationship between energy utilization, cell signaling, and life span. The suggestion that a shift in metabolic pathways that can be triggered by several cues, such as caloric restriction and nutrient sensing, is intriguing when considered alongside the chapters dealing with longevity in mammals. Do such metabolic shifts underlie the hormetic response that is suggested by Drs. Matzko and company and are they at play in the long-lived animals described by Brown–Borg et al.? In a larger context, the balance that is struck between energy intake and fecundity is consistent with evolutionary theories of aging *(7, 8)*.

Examples of the third category of pathways that appear to modulate changes in life span/aging include those involved in DNA damage repair, cell cycle checkpoints, senescence, and apoptosis. These fundamental cellular mechanisms would not be predicted to vary greatly in response to immediate environmental influences, yet they are widely believed to be important in aging. The evidence that genomic integrity is important to aging and life span depends primarily on the reduction in life span and rapid senescence phenotypes that result from mutations in proteins involved in genomic maintenance. Werner's syndrome is an excellent example of a mutation, in this case a DNA helicase, involved with DNA damage response and genome stability, and ultimately important for life span *(9)*. Other examples include the accelerated aging caused by a reduction in the levels of Ku 80, a protein critical to nonhomologous end joining *(10)* or increased activity of p53 *(11)*. This third category of pathways may be less responsive to environmental influences than are the first two categories and is part of the cellular maintenance mechanism that is required for normal life span.

## 3 Environmental Pressures That Modulate Life Span

The external triggers that induce the responses outlined above are numerous. Experimentally, stresses such as low nutrient availability and mild stresses such as heat shock or low-level radiation in *D. melanogaster* are paradigms for extending life span. Dr. Longo shows that blunting the intracellular pathways central to nutrient sensing can lead to life-span extension in yeast that are in a stable, growth-arrested state. Similar pathways seem to be involved in the response of mice to caloric restriction but, as would be expected in a multicellular organism, the response is multifaceted. The complexity of the response to caloric restriction in rodents and its relationship to response to stress are explored in the chapter by Matzko, McCarter, and Masoro. The overall picture that seems to emerge is that population life span is influenced by stress responses that can be influenced by a number of external signals and act through a set of conserved intracellular pathways. One intriguing question is the nature of the relationship of these responses, if any, to species life span. We would predict that species life span is molded by response to environmental influences resulting in the establishment of an aging trajectory that is characteristic for a given species. The mechanisms that drive this process and their relationship to the interventional studies that modulate life span in a specific species and experimental setting are, however, unclear. The chapters contributed by Dr. Buffenstein deal with a comparative approach to aging that seeks to address these questions. Specifically, what are the fundamental mechanisms that lead to species-specific differences in life span? The difficult task of identifying these mechanisms requires the type of comparative analysis involving animals such as the extraordinary naked mole-rat. These models, combined with the advent of more advanced techniques for comparative analysis, will provide information regarding these mechanisms.

In summary, the field of aging is expanding exponentially with extraordinary advances coming from multiple approaches. We hope that the collection of viewpoints assembled here will provide insight and food for thought to those interested in this area.

**Acknowledgments** We sincerely thank all the authors for their wonderful contributions and patience during the production process. Finally, we thank Pam Fried and Diana Winters for their tireless work in copyediting the manuscripts.

## References

1. Lithgow GJ. Why aging isn't regulated: A lamentation on the use of language in aging literature. Exp Gerontol 2006;41:890–3.
2. Butler RN, Warner HR, Williams TF, et al. The aging factor in health and disease: the promise of basic research on aging. Aging Clin Exp Res 2004;16:104–11; discussion 11–2.
3. Warner H, Anderson J, Austad S, et al. Science fact and the SENS agenda. What can we reasonably expect from ageing research? EMBO Rep 2005;6:1006–8.
4. Muller FL, Lustgarten MS, Jang Y, Richardson A, Van Remmen H. Trends in oxidative aging theories. Free Radic Biol Med 2007;43:477–503.
5. Nebert DW, Dalton TP. The role of cytochrome P450 enzymes in endogenous signalling pathways and environmental carcinogenesis. Nat Rev Cancer 2006;6:947–60.
6. Amador-Noguez D, Dean A, Huang W, Setchell K, Moore D, Darlington G. Alterations in xenobiotic metabolism in the long-lived Little mice. Aging Cell 2007;6:453–70.
7. Kirkwood TB, Austad SN. Why do we age? Nature 2000;408:233–8.
8. Hughes KA, Reynolds RM. Evolutionary and mechanistic theories of aging. Annu Rev Entomol 2005;50:421–45.
9. Kudlow BA, Kennedy BK, Monnat RJ, Jr. Werner and Hutchinson-Gilford progeria syndromes: Mechanistic basis of human progeroid diseases. Nat Rev Mol Cell Biol 2007;8:394–404.
10. Li H, Vogel H, Holcomb VB, Gu Y, Hasty P. Deletion of Ku70, Ku80, or both causes early aging without substantially increased cancer. Mol Cell Biol 2007;27:8205–14.
11. Campisi J. Aging and cancer cell biology. Aging Cell 2008;7:281–4.

# Part I
# Yeast

# Chapter 1
# Reprogramming Cell Survival and Longevity: The Role of Tor, Sch9, Ras, and Sir2

**Valter D. Longo**

**Abstract** *Saccharomyces cerevisiae* has emerged as the simplest of the major model systems to study cell survival and aging. Among the key proteins that regulate aging in this unicellular eukaryote are Tor/Sch9, Ras, and Sir2. Remarkably, similar genes and pathways are implicated in the regulation of longevity in worms, flies, and mice, suggesting that the "test-tube" approach can provide fundamental clues to understand how mammalian cells survive and die during normal aging. The role of Tor/Sch9, Ras, and Sir2 in reprogramming survival and chronological life span in *S. cerevisiae* and their potentially conserved role in higher eukaryotes are reviewed.

**Keywords** Ras • Akt • Sch9 • Sir2 • life span • aging • yeast

**Abbreviations** AC: Adenylyl cyclase; CFU: Colony forming unit; ERCs: Extra-chromosomal ribosomal DNA circles; FOXO: Forkhead; GH: Growth hormone; IGF-I: Insulin-like growth factor I; PKA: Protein kinase A; PKB: Protein kinase B; SDC: Synthetic dextrose complete; YPD: Yeast extract, peptone, dextrose

## 1.1 Introduction

Our understanding of the fundamental mechanisms and genetics of aging has relied primarily on studies in *Saccharomyces cerevisiae*, *Caenorhabditis elegans*, *Drosophila melanogaster*, and *Mus musculus*. The discovery that aging in these

V.D. Longo
Andrus Gerontology Center and Department of Biological Sciences,
University of Southern California, Los Angeles, CA, 90089-0191, USA
e-mail: vlongo@usc.edu

C. Sell et al. (eds.), *Life-Span Extension,* Aging Medicine,
DOI 10.1007/978-1-60327-507-1_1,

organisms is regulated by a conserved set of genes implicated in a variety of diseases ***(1–3)*** may represent "the end of the beginning" of the research on aging ***(4)***. Yeast is a particularly valuable model organism for aging studies because of its relatively short life span, the straightforward genetic techniques available, and the high-throughput technologies recently developed specifically for this unicellular eukaryote. Notably, *S. cerevisiae* is both a cell and an organism. Thus, it is a useful system to study the fundamental mechanisms of aging that occur in more complex organisms but also in both dividing and nondividing mammalian cells.

The yeast replicative life span, measured by counting the number of buds produced by individual mother cells (replicative or budding life span) ***(5, 6)***, can serve as a model system for mammalian cells undergoing replicative aging, whereas yeast aging chronologically in a nondividing survival phase (chronological life span) models aging in higher eukaryotes but also in both dividing and nondividing mammalian cells ***(7)***. In fact, chronologically aging yeast cells do not divide but maintain the ability to divide for the majority of their life span ***(8)***. *C. elegans* represents the second simplest and perhaps the more widely studied model system for aging ***(9)***. Being made up of only about 1,000 somatic cells, it provides both the advantages of a multicellular organism and those of a relatively simple genetic system, although it is less amenable than *S. cerevisiae* to biochemical studies. Thus, *C. elegans* together with *D. melanogaster* provides a link between the molecular studies in yeast and studies in mammalian cells. The fourth major model system, the long-lived mouse (30 months and more) *M. musculus*, has the disadvantage of being much more complex and difficult to study, but it is obviously an essential system because of its much closer phylogenetic relationship to humans.

The genetics of aging in yeast with a focus on the genes that affect the chronological life span is reviewed. The similarities between the genes and pathways that regulate survival in yeast, worms, flies, and mice with emphasis on Ras, Akt, and Sir2 are also discussed.

## 1.2 The *S. cerevisiae* Chronological Life Span

Microorganisms have evolved to survive under adverse conditions that are commonly encountered in the wild. In fact, most microorganisms are estimated to survive in a low-metabolism stationary phase under conditions of limited nutrients ***(10)***. In the wild, yeast organisms are likely to exit the stationary phase only during the rare periods when all the nutrients required for growth become available. A common misconception is that chronological survival in the postdiauxic (postswitch from fermentable to nonfermentable carbon sources) and stationary phases only models starvation conditions in higher eukaryotes. In fact, the DBY746 wild-type cells grown in 2% glucose synthetic dextrose complete (SDC) medium maintain high levels of ethanol and other nutrients in the extracellular medium for the entire survival period

*(11)*. Furthermore, *S. cerevisiae* stores glycogen and other nutrients required for survival intracellularly *(12)*, and incubation in water increases chronological survival *(13)*. Yeast grown and incubated in the nutrient-rich yeast extract, peptone, dextrose (YPD) medium also survives for months in a low-metabolism stationary phase. However, it is not clear whether YPD medium allows some growth to occur during the apparently stationary phase.

In addition to the high-metabolism postdiauxic life span and the low-metabolism stationary phase, under particularly severe starvation conditions, diploid *S. cerevisiae* can form haploid spores that may survive for years in a dormant state. The yeast spore resembles the very long-lived worm dauer larva, entered at the L2 larva stage during periods of starvation *(14)*. However, most yeast diploid organisms enter and remain in the stationary phase, and only a minority of diploid organisms form spores *(15)*. Most of the chronological life-span studies are performed using haploid strains, which behave similarly to diploid cells under most conditions but do not sporulate.

## 1.3 High-Metabolism Survival in Synthetic Dextrose Complete Medium

Chronological life-span studies are normally performed by monitoring survival in the high-metabolism postdiauxic phase entered by cells grown in SDC medium, which contains glucose, yeast nitrogen base, agar, ammonium sulfate (nitrogen source), sodium phosphate, vitamins, metals, and salts. After approximately 10 h of exponential growth at 30°C in shaking flasks, the glucose concentration in the medium reaches very low levels, and yeast switch from a fermentation- to a respiration-based metabolism. During fermentative growth, ethanol is accumulated and released from the cells *(11)*. In wild-type DBY746 and SP1 cultures, the level of ethanol undergoes an age-dependent decline, but it is not depleted, suggesting that it is used as a carbon source for the entire life span. When yeast organisms are incubated in SDC, the diauxic shift is followed by a postdiauxic phase, in which some growth continues slowly until approximately 48–72 h, when the final density reached is about 100 million cells/ml (Fig. 1.1). In this phase, metabolic rates remain high until day 4–6 and then decrease at least tenfold. The mean survival time of wild-type strains depends on their genetic background; it ranges from 6–7 days for the DBY746 or SP1 wild-type cells to 15–20 days for S288C or BY4700 wild-type cells.

In a standard postdiauxic experiment, survival is monitored by measuring the ability of an individual yeast cell or organism to form a colony (colony forming unit [CFU]) within 3 days of plating onto rich medium plates. CFUs are normally monitored until at least 99.9% of the population dies. The number of CFUs at day 3 is considered to be the initial survival rate (100% survival) and is used to determine the age-dependent survival rate. The correlation between the loss of CFUs and

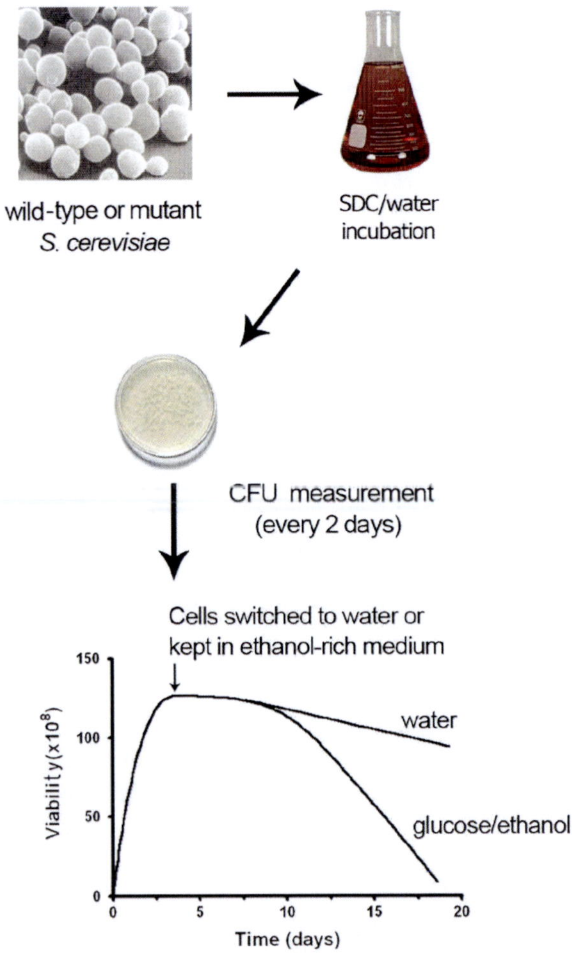


**Fig. 1.1** Populations of wild-type or mutant yeast are grown in minimal medium containing glucose (SDC). After 2 to 3 days, cell growth stops and ethanol accumulates in the medium. At day 3 yeast are either kept in this ethanol-rich medium or switched to water. Cell viability is measured every 2 days by diluting the yeast cultures and plating an appropriate number of cells onto rich medium (YPD) plates to monitor the colony forming units (CFUs). When yeast are switched to water, the cultures are washed every 2 days to avoid the cell division that might be caused by the accumulation of nutrients released from the dead yeast

death has been confirmed by a live–dead fluorescence assay to monitor the percentage of live cells over time. After staining a sample of cells with the FUN-1 dye, which confers red fluorescence to live cells and green–yellow fluorescence to dead cells, the live:dead ratio was found to be consistent with the CFU-based viability data *(8)*. The age-dependent increase in the level of proteins released from dead cells into the medium is also consistent with the CFU and live–dead data *(8)*.

## 1.4 Severe Calorie Restriction: Survival in Water

The reduction of calories by 30–50% or more has been shown to extend the life span of many organisms ***(16)***. As mentioned earlier, *S. cerevisiae* switched from glucose/ethanol-containing medium to water survive much longer (see Fig. 1.1). In fact, the mean life span of strains DBY746 and SP1 in water is 2–3 times longer than in SDC (15–20 days). Incubation in water can also rule out the possibility that the extended life span of a particular mutant is an artifact caused by regrowth in the liquid cultures. In fact, after more than 99% of wild-type DBY746 and SP1 yeast incubated in SDC dies, in about 50% of the studies, a better-adapted subpopulation is able to grow back by utilizing the nutrients released by dead cells ***(17)***. A similar phenomenon called "gasping" is observed for populations of bacteria ***(18)***. Such growth creates a mixed population containing both young and old organisms, which invalidates the survival studies.

For life-span studies in water, yeast are grown in SDC medium and incubated for 3 days, washed with sterile distilled water, and resuspended in sterile water (see Fig. 1.1). Viability is monitored by measuring CFUs every 2 days. The cells are washed three times with water every 2 days to minimize the chance of growth during long-term survival in the stationary phase *(7)*.

## 1.5 Yeast Replicative Life Span

The asymmetrical division characteristic of *S. cerevisiae* allows the measurement of the replicative life span. Daughter cells are normally smaller than mother cells and can be easily distinguished and removed from their progenitors by micromanipulation ***(6)***. The average replicative life span is approximately 20 divisions in the DBY746 wild-type background but varies greatly in other backgrounds. Aged cells divide more slowly and become sterile. When cell division stops, they are counted as dead, although their postreproductive survival time is poorly understood ***(19)***. Although few genes are known to regulate both life spans, the relationship between replicative and chronological aging has yet to be established. Notably, yeast replicative life span is analogous to the replicative life span of mammalian fibroblasts and lymphocytes, which undergo a limited number of population doublings in culture. Thus, the "budding life span" is a model to study aging of mitotic cells, but it can also provide insights into the fundamental mechanisms of organismal aging.

Replicative aging can be caused by a form of genomic instability that leads to the accumulation of extrachromosomal ribosomal DNA circles (ERCs) ***(20)*** and is delayed by increasing the activity of the silencing regulator Sir2 ***(21)***. Sir2 is an NAD-dependent histone deacetylase whose activity is required to promote chromatin silencing at the telomeres, mating type loci, and rDNA ***(22, 23)***. Increased dosage of *SIR2* delays replicative aging by inhibiting rDNA recombination and consequently the formation of ERCs *(21)*. Although this aging mechanism has not been observed in any other species, Sir2 was shown to play a conserved antiaging role in higher eukaryotes.

## 1.6 Evolutionarily Conserved Proaging Pathways

Other genes implicated in the regulation of replicative aging have been identified. Among these are *RAS1/RAS2* and *LAG1/LAG2*. *RAS1* and *RAS2* play opposite roles in replicative aging. The deletion of *RAS1* extends replicative life span. By contrast, lack of *RAS2* shortens replicative longevity ***(24)***. Intriguingly, lack of *RAS2* promotes chronological survival ***(8, 25)***. Overexpression of Lag1, a protein implicated in ceramide synthesis, extends replicative life span ***(26)***. The activation of the retrograde response also triggers replicative life-span extension. This response is activated by an intracellular signaling pathway from the mitochondrion to the nucleus and leads to the transcription of several genes encoding for metabolic enzymes ***(27)***.

The serine/threonine kinase Tor/Sch9 and Tor have been shown to block the effect of calorie restriction on the extension of the *S. cerevisiae* replicative life span ***(28)***, confirming that the chronological and replicative life spans of yeast are regulated by overlapping mechanisms.

## 1.7 The Genetics of Chronological Aging: Reprogramming Stress Resistance and Cell Survival

Using the chronological aging paradigm, our laboratory and others have identified several mutations that promote life-span extension and resistance to both heat and oxidative stress. Among these is the deletion of the gene coding for the serine/threonine kinase Sch9. Lack of Sch9 promotes resistance to high stress and extends the life span up to threefold ***(29)***. Reduced Tor activity also extends the chronological life span ***(30, 31)***. Our results suggest that Tor and Sch9 are likely to function in the same longevity regulatory pathway. Tor/Sch9 are part of a glucose-sensing pathway that regulates cell division, cell size, ribosomal synthesis, and the expression of stress resistance proteins including mitochondrial superoxide dismutase (Sod2) ***(8, 32–34)***. Importantly, Sch9 is homologous to Akt/protein kinase B (PKB) and S6 kinase, components of the conserved proaging pathways of worms, flies, and possibly mice (see Sect. 1.4) ***(35)*** (Fig. 1.2). Another glucose-sensing pathway known to regulate chronological aging is the Cyr1/Ras/protein kinase A (PKA) pathway. The reduced activity of adenylate cyclase (Cyr1) promotes stress resistance and longevity and so does the deletion of *RAS2*, which encodes for a highly conserved progrowth signaling

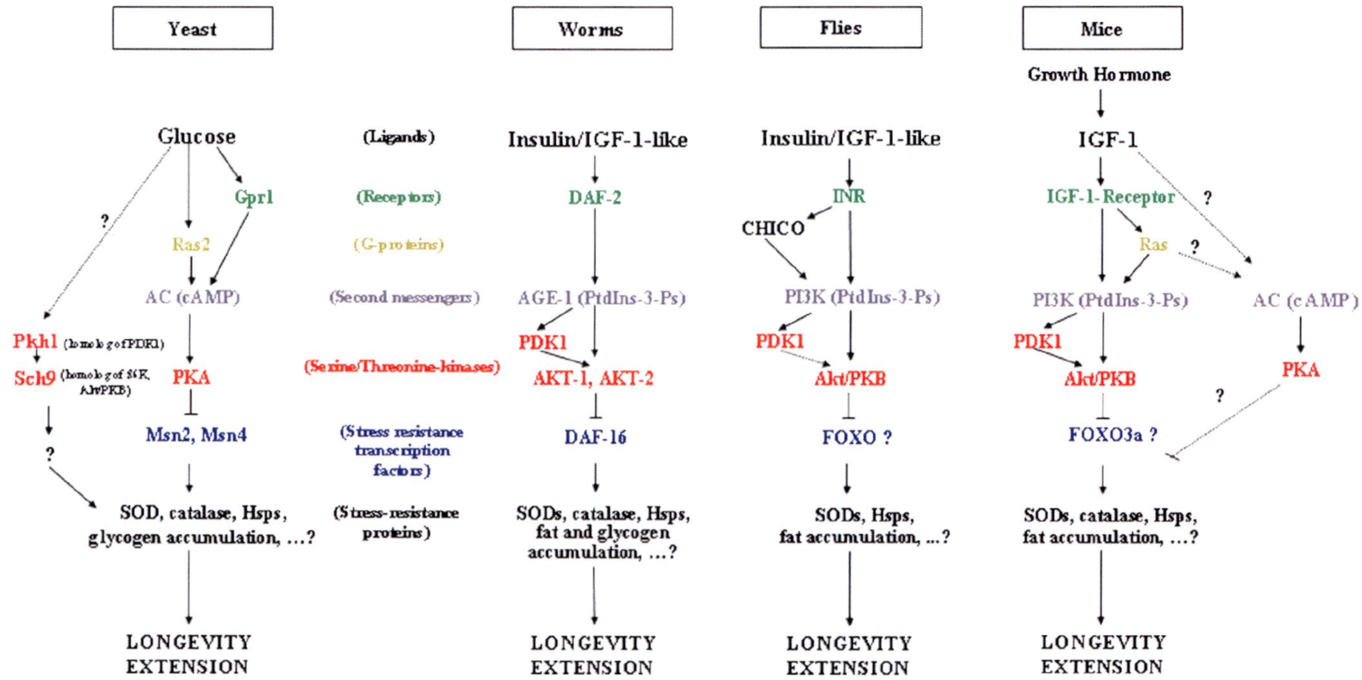


**Fig. 1.2** Conserved regulation of longevity. In yeast, worms, flies, and mice the downregulation of partially conserved glucose or insulin/insulin-like growth factor I (IGF-I) promotes the expression of antioxidant enzymes and heat-shock proteins, induces the accumulation of glycogen or fat, and extends life span. In yeast and worms the induction of stress resistance is required for longevity extension. In flies and mice a conclusive role for stress resistance induction in promoting life span has not been established yet. Tor/Sch9 and Pkh1 are functional homologues of Akt1 and PDK1, respectively

G-protein *(8, 25, 29)*. Although the adenylate cyclase/PKA pathway has not been implicated in life-span regulation in worms and flies, a recent study suggests that, analogous to the results in yeast, the downregulation of the adenylate cyclase/PKA pathway by deletion of 5 adenylyl cyclase (AC5) extends the life span of mice and protects them from reduced bone density and aging-induced cardiomyopathy *(36)*. The downregulation of the Ras/AC/PKA pathway promotes chronological survival via the activation of stress resistance transcription factors Msn2/Msn4 *(29)*, which in turn activate the expression of the detoxifying enzymes catalase and superoxide dismutase and of several heat-shock proteins *(37–39)* (see Fig. 1.2). Reduced Ras/AC/PKA activity also promotes the accumulation of reserve carbohydrate glycogen. The yeast Tor/Sch9 and Ras/AC/PKA pathways share several gene targets, although in some cases their regulation of gene expression is opposite *(40)*. The exact relationship between these two pathways is still unclear, mainly because the pathway components upstream and downstream of Sch9 have been elusive. A recent in vitro study showed that the protein kinase Pkh1 can phosphorylate and activate Sch9 and that this activation is stimulated by phytosphingosine *(41)*. This finding is important because Pkh1 is a yeast homolog of PDK1, a protein also found in the proaging insulin/insulin-like growth factor I (IGF-I) pathways of worms, flies, and mice. Tor was also recently shown to phosphorylate and regulate Sch9 *(42)*, supporting the possibility that Tor and Sch9 function in the same aging regulatory pathway. These data are also in agreement with the hypothesis that the yeast pathway including Tor, Pkh1, and Sch9 and the mouse pathway including insulin/IGF-I, Tor, PDK1/2, AKT, and S6K originated from a common ancestral pathway (see Fig. 1.2).

The ability to withstand oxidative stress is one of the conserved features of long-lived mutants. We have shown that manganese superoxide dismutase functions as a mediator of longevity extension in both the Ras and Tor/Sch9 pathways and is required for chronological longevity extension *(8)*. In fact, the tricarboxylic acid cycle enzyme aconitase is a key target of mitochondrial superoxide toxicity, and loss of aconitase activity precedes death in yeast aging chronologically *(8, 29)*. Analogous to our findings in yeast, AC5-deficient mice showed increased levels of manganese superoxide dismutase and stress resistance *(36)*.

The activity of the Hsp90 chaperone also affects chronological survival. Reducing the activity of Hsp82, one of the yeast Hsp90 proteins, extends the chronological life span by overactivating the heat-shock transcription factor HSF1 and consequently the heat-shock response *(43)*. Further genes involved in the regulation of chronological aging are *YAP1*, *YCA1*, and *AIF1*. Overexpression of *YAP1*, which encodes for an oxygen stress response transcription factor, reduces the accumulation of reactive oxygen species during chronological aging and promotes life-span extension *(44)*. Deletion of either *YCA1*, coding for a yeast caspase, or *AIF1*, coding for a homolog of the mammalian apoptosis-inducing factor, extends chronological survival *(45, 46)*.

## 1.8 Sir2 and Yeast Chronological Aging

The role of Sir2 in the chronological survival of nondividing yeast cells has only recently been examined ***(47)*** and appears to be quite different from its role in the yeast replicative life span. Deletion of *SIR2* has no effect on the chronological life span of wild-type yeast but extends further the chronological life span of mutants with reduced PKA or Tor/Sch9 activity (Fig. 1.3) ***(47)***. Other sirtuins have not been examined in this aging assay. Evidence exists for two possible mechanisms by which deletion of *SIR2* results in life-span extension when coupled with reduced nutrient-responsive kinase activity. First, deletion of *SIR2* in combination with reduced PKA or Sch9 activity was found to decrease the rate of DNA mutations that accumulate with age in postmitotic conditions ***(47)***. This finding is in contrast with the role of Sir2 in mitotically active cells, in which it promotes genome stability by repressing recombination ***(48)***. Second, *sir2Δ* cells have elevated levels of the alcohol dehydrogenase Adh2 (see Fig. 1.3) ***(47)***. Mitotically active yeast cells generate energy primarily through fermentation, leading to the production of ethanol. As fermentable carbon sources become scarce and ethanol accumulates, yeast undergo a metabolic shift and begin to use ethanol as an energy source, only entering the stationary phase after ethanol levels are largely depleted. In the absence of Sir2, increased alcohol dehydrogenase activity leads to more rapid ethanol degradation and entry into a

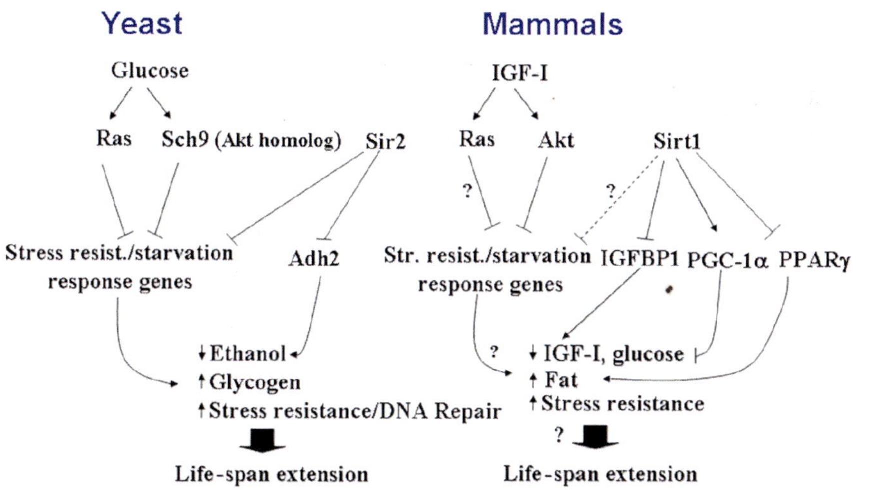


**Fig. 1.3** Models for life-span extension by reduced Sir2 function. In the yeast chronological life-span assay, deletion of *SIR2* has been shown to enhance survival in a postmitotic state either in low nutrient conditions or when combined with mutations in nutrient-responsive kinases such as Ras, Sch9, and TOR. *sir2Δ* strains show elevated stress resistance and enhanced alcohol dehydrogenase activity under these conditions, although the mechanisms by which Sir2 regulates these processes remain largely to be determined. In mammals, the longevity effects of Sirt1 have not been reported. However, Sirt1 is reported to have a number of functions that may regulate longevity

more stable postmitotic state. The mechanism by which Sir2 negatively regulates Adh2 levels as cells enter a postmitotic state has yet to be determined.

## 1.9 Evolutionary Conserved Proaging Pathways

Similar proaging pathways have been identified in all aging-model organisms, suggesting that a strategy to regulate life span may have appeared early during evolution ***(1, 3)*** (Figs. 1.2 and 1.4). As described earlier, two glucose-sensing pathways are central regulators of chronological aging in yeast: the Tor/Sch9 and the Ras/PKA pathways (see Fig. 1.2). Research conducted in *C. elegans* has identified the insulin/IGF-I-like pathway as a major proaging pathway (see Fig. 1.2). The similarities between yeast- and worm-aging pathways are remarkable. Analogous to the yeast Ras/PKA and Tor/Sch9 pathways, the insulin/IGF-I-like pathway senses the presence of nutrients and regulates entry into a hypometabolic stage (dauer larva). Worm life span can be extended up to three times by reducing the activity of some of the components of the insulin/IGF-I-like pathway such as the cellular receptor DAF-2 and PI-3 kinase AGE-1 ***(9, 49–52)***. Importantly, AGE-1 activates kinase Akt/PKB, which is homologous to yeast Sch9 and can also be activated by PDK-1, the homolog of yeast Pkh1 (see Fig. 1.2) ***(51)***. Life-span extension in both daf-2 and age-1 mutants requires the activity of stress resistance transcription factor DAF-16, which belongs to the forkhead (FOXO) family of transcription factors, and of the heat-shock transcription factor HSF-1, a highly conserved heat-shock protein ***(52, 53)***. The mediators of longevity extension downstream of DAF-16 are also partially conserved between yeast and worms and include mitochondrial superoxide dismutase, catalase, and several heat-shock proteins (see Fig. 1.2). Long-lived mutants of both species store carbon in the form of glycogen (yeast and worm) or fat (worm).

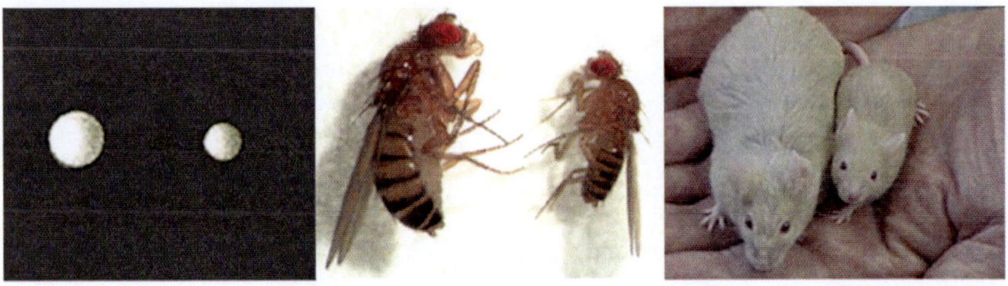

**Fig. 1.4** Yeast, flies, and mice with mutations that decrease glucose or insulin/IGF-I-like signaling. Wild-type (*left*) and long-lived dwarf (*right*) yeast; yeast *sch9Δ* null mutants form smaller colonies (*left panel*; from [3], reprinted with permission from AAAS). *sch9Δ* mutants are also smaller in size, grow at a slower rate, and survive three times longer than wild-type yeast. *Chico* homozygous mutant female flies are dwarf animals and exhibit an increase in life span of up to 50% (*center panel*) (figure provided by D. Gems). *Chico* functions in the fly insulin/IGF-I-like signaling pathway. The GHR/BP mice are dwarf animals deficient in IGF-I and exhibit a 50% increase in life span (*right panel*) (figure provided by A. Bartke; photo by Michael Bonkowski). Other yeast and worm mutants exhibit life-span extension of more than 100% but do not have detectable growth defects (see text)

The insulin-IGF-I pathway has also been linked to the regulation of aging in *Drosophila* (see Figs. 1.2 and 1.4). Reducing the activity of this pathway by mutating the insulin receptor or the insulin receptor substrate (*chico*) extends the life span of the fruit fly by up to 85%. This life-span extension is associated with increased levels of superoxide dismutase activity and fat accumulation (see Fig. 1.2) ***(54, 55)***. Notably, as shown in yeast, the mitochondrial enzyme aconitase is oxidatively modified and inactivated in old flies ***(56)***. Thus, impairing mitochondrial respiration by inactivating aconitase appears to be an age-dependent phenomenon shared between species and increasing superoxide dismutase activity, a common mechanism that contributes to longevity extension. In fact, overexpression of *SOD1/SOD2* in yeast and flies causes a modest but significant extension of life span ***(8, 57–59)***. The life span of *Drosophila* is also extended by overexpressing dFOXO, a homolog of the worm DAF-16, in the peripheral fat body ***(60, 61)***.

Mammals have separate receptors for IGF-I and insulin. Research in mice has connected both receptors to life-span regulation. Dwarf mice with a defective pituitary gland and consequently deficient in growth hormone (GH) and IGF-I live up to 65% longer than wild-type mice and are stress resistant ***(62, 63)*** (see Figs. 1.2 and 1.4). The effect of dwarf mutations on life span appears to be caused by reduction in GH and IGF-I signaling because mice lacking the GH receptor are long lived ***(64)*** and IGF-I receptor heterozygous knockout mice live 30% longer than wild type ***(65)***. Furthermore, mice lacking the insulin receptor in the adipose tissue live 18% longer than wild-type mice ***(66)***. Stress resistance also appears to be regulated by GH and IGF-I. In fact, the activities of superoxide dismutases and catalase are decreased after exposure of murine hepatocytes to GH or IGF-I and in transgenic mice overexpressing GH ***(67, 68)***. Like the worm daf-2 and the fly *InR* mutants, dwarf mice accumulate fat, suggesting that the accumulation of reserve carbon sources is an important and conserved portion of a maintenance mode aimed at slowing down aging and surviving through periods of starvation. Analogously, long-lived yeast mutants accumulate glycogen, their main reserve carbon source during starvation. Mammalian FOXO transcription factors, homologs of the life-span extending DAF-16 and dFOXO transcription factors, have not been conclusively linked with life-span regulation in mammals. However, FOXO activity is associated with increased stress resistance and elevated mitochondrial superoxide dismutase activity in quiescent cells (see Fig. 1.2) ***(69)***.

As shown for *S. cerevisiae*, increased dosage of the Sir2 homologues extends the life span of both *C. elegans* and *Drosophila* by up to 50%, and Sir2 activity has been associated with the longevity extension caused by calorie restriction, an intervention known to extend the life span of all model organisms ***(70–72)***. As described earlier, yeast Sir2 also plays a proaging role in combination with mutations in the *RAS* or TOR/SCH9 pathway ***(11)***. Sir2 may play a similar proaging role in *C. elegans* because its deletion increases further the life span of the very long-lived DAF-2 mutants ***(73)***. Despite the extensive experimental efforts to link the Sir2 family of proteins (sirtuins) to mammalian longevity, a conclusive role for the sirtuins in mediating life-span regulation has yet to be established.

## 1.10 Conclusions

Studies in *S. cerevisiae*, *C. elegans*, *Drosophila*, and mice have resulted in the identification of many genes and of a few conserved pathways that can be activated or inactivated to extend the life span of the cell or organism. The role of these antiaging pathways in the regulation of stress resistance, the storage of reserve carbon sources, and the expression of many genes involved in virtually every aspect of cell function suggest that they are the central unit of a "survival or longevity program." Tor, Sch9, Ras2, and various stress resistance transcription factors have emerged as major mediators of this program in yeast but also in worms, flies, and mice. The Ras/AC/PKA pathway promotes aging in yeast, but, although Ras functions downstream of the IGF-I receptor in mammals and is implicated in cell death, it has not been shown to regulate aging in higher eukaryotes. However, recent results indicate that AC5 and PKA promote aging and diseases in mice ***(36)***.

The partial conservation of the regulation of survival extension from yeast to mammals together with the availability of characterization studies on the majority of *S. cerevisiae* proteins makes this unicellular eukaryote the simplest and one of the most valuable model systems in which to study the fundamental mechanisms of aging. Yeast and higher eukaryotes appear to use similar "molecular strategies" to regulate entry into maintenance phases that extend life span. These strategies, which include downregulation of glucose- or IGF-I-like receptor-activated signal transduction proteins, activation of stress resistance transcription factors, upregulation of antioxidant enzymes and heat-shock proteins, and increased storage of reserve nutrients, are also likely to extend to many additional biological processes including repair and replacement systems. We predict that we will continue to observe some difference but many fundamental similarities between these longevity regulatory pathways in eukaryotes. An important aim should be to begin to apply the knowledge of these powerful, conserved antiaging pathways to human diseases. Whereas modern medicine is focused on the treatment of diseases, the identification of conserved antiaging genes and pathways should eventually provide a novel "evolutionary medicine" approach in which multiple diseases of aging, including cancer, Alzheimer, and cardiovascular diseases, can be prevented by redistributing energy from reproduction and growth to maintenance and consequently extending the cell survival and organismal longevity program.

**Acknowledgments** Related work in the laboratory of VDL is supported by American Federation for Aging Research ***(74)*** grant (P.F.) and by NIH AG20642 and AG01028.

## References

1. Kenyon C. A conserved regulatory system for aging. Cell 2001;105:165–8.
2. Longo VD. Mutations in signal transduction proteins increase stress resistance and longevity in yeast, nematodes, fruit flies, and mammalian neuronal cells. Neurobiol Aging 1999;20:479–86.

3. Longo VD, Finch CE. Evolutionary medicine: from dwarf model systems to healthy centenarians. Science 2003;299:1342–6.
4. Martin GM, LaMarco K, Strauss E, Kelner K. Research on aging: the end of the beginning. Science 2003;299:1339–41.
5. Jazwinski SM, Egilmez NK, Chen JB. Replication control and cellular life span. Exp Gerontol 1989;24:423–36.
6. Mortimer RK. Life span of individual yeast cells. Nature 1959;183:1751–2.
7. Fabrizio P, Longo VD. The chronological life span of Saccharomyces cerevisiae. Aging Cell 2003;2:73–81.
8. Fabrizio P, Liou LL, Moy VN, Diaspro A, et al. SOD2 functions downstream of Sch9 to extend longevity in yeast. Genetics 2003;163:35–46.
9. Johnson TE. Aging can be genetically dissected into component processes using long-lived lines of *Caenorhabditis elegans*. Proc Natl Acad Sci U S A 1987;84:3777–81.
10. Werner-Washburne M, Braun EL, Crawford ME, Peck VM. Stationary phase in *Saccharomyces cerevisiae*. Mol Microbiol 1986;19:1159–66.
11. Fabrizio P, Gattazzo C, Battistella L, et al. Sir2 blocks extreme life-span extension [see comment]. Cell 2005;123:655–7.
12. Lillie SH, Pringle JR. Reserve carbohydrate metabolism in *Saccharomyces cerevisiae:* response to nutrient limitation. J Bacteriol 1980;143:1384–94.
13. Longo VD, Ellerby LM, Bredesen DE, Valentine JS, Gralla EB. Human Bcl-2 reverses survival defects in yeast lacking superoxide dismutase and delays death of wild-type yeast. J Cell Biol 1997;137:1581–8.
14. Riddle DL. The nematode *C. elegans*. Cold Spring Harbor, NY: Cold Spring Harbor Laboratory Press, 1988.
15. Codon AC, Gasent-Ramirez JM, Benitez T. Factors which affect the frequency of sporulation and tetrad formation in *Saccharomyces cerevisiae* baker's yeasts [published erratum appears in Appl Environ Microbiol 1995;61:1677]. Appl Environ Microbiol 1995;61: 630–8.
16. Sohal RS, Weindruch R. Oxidative stress, caloric restriction, and aging. Science 1996;273:59–63.
17. Fabrizio P, Battistella L, Vardavas R, et al. Superoxide is a mediator of an altruistic aging program in *Saccharomyces cerevisiae*. J Cell Biol 2004;166:1055–67.
18. Zambrano MM, Kolter R. GASPing for life in stationary phase. Cell 1996;86:181–4.
19. Bitterman KJ, Medvedik O, Sinclair DA. Longevity regulation in *Saccharomyces cerevisiae*: linking metabolism, genome stability, and heterochromatin. Microbiol Mol Biol Rev 2003;67:376–99.
20. Sinclair DA, Guarente L. Extrachromosomal rDNA circles: a cause of aging in yeast. Cell 1997;91:1033–42.
21. Kaeberlein M, McVey M, Guarente L. The SIR2/3/4 complex and SIR2 alone promote longevity in *Saccharomyces cerevisiae* by two different mechanisms. Genes Dev 1999;13:2570–80.
22. Braunstein M, Rose AB, Holmes SG, Allis CD, Broach JR. Transcriptional silencing in yeast is associated with reduced nucleosome acetylation. Genes Dev 1993;7:592–604.
23. Tanny JC, Dowd GJ, Huang J, Hilz H, Moazed D. An enzymatic activity in the yeast Sir2 protein that is essential for gene silencing. Cell 1999;99:735–45.
24. Sun J, Kale SP, Childress AM, Pinswasdi C, Jazwinski SM. Divergent roles of RAS1 and RAS2 in yeast longevity. J Biol Chem 1994;269:18638–45.
25. Longo VD. The pro-senescence role of Ras2 in the chronological life span of yeast [thesis]. Los Angeles, CA: University of California Los Angeles, 1997.
26. D'Mello NP, Childress AM, Franklin DS, Kale SP, Pinswasdi C, Jazwinski SM. Cloning and characterization of LAG1, a longevity-assurance gene in yeast. J Biol Chem 1994;269:15451–9.
27. Kirchman PA, Kim S, Lai CY, Jazwinski SM. Interorganelle signaling is a determinant of longevity in *Saccharomyces cerevisiae*. Genetics 1999;152:179–90.

28. Kaeberlein M, Powers RW III, Steffen KK, et al. Regulation of yeast replicative life span by TOR and Sch9 in response to nutrients [see comment]. Science 2005;310:1193–6.
29. Fabrizio P, Pozza F, Pletcher SD, Gendron CM, Longo VD. Regulation of longevity and stress resistance by Sch9 in yeast. Science 2001;292:288–90.
30. Powers RW III, Kaeberlein M, Caldwell SD, Kennedy BK, Fields S. Extension of chronological life span in yeast by decreased TOR pathway signaling. Genes Dev 2006;20:174–84.
31. Wei M, Fabrizio P, Hu J, Ge H, Cheng C, Li L, Longo VD. Life span extension by calorie restriction depends on Rim15 and transcription factors downstream of Ras/PKA, Tor, and Sch9. PLoS Genet 2008;4:e13.
32. Jorgensen P, Nishikawa JL, Breitkreutz BJ, Tyers M. Systematic identification of pathways that couple cell growth and division in yeast. Science 2002;297:395–400.
33. Jorgensen P, Rupes I, Sharom JR, Schneper L, Broach JR, Tyers M. A dynamic transcriptional network communicates growth potential to ribosome synthesis and critical cell size. Genes Dev 2004;18:2491–505.
34. Toda T, Cameron S, Sass P, Wigler M. SCH9, a gene of *Saccharomyces cerevisiae* that encodes a protein distinct from, but functionally and structurally related to, cAMP-dependent protein kinase catalytic subunits. Genes Dev 1988;2:517–27.
35. Geyskens I, Kumara S, Donaton M, Bergsma J, Thevelein J, Wera S. Expression of mammalian PKB complements deletion of the yeast protein kinase Sch9. NATO ASI Ser A, Life Sci 2000;A316:117–26.
36. Yan L, Vatner DE, O'Connor JP, et al. Type 5 adenylyl cyclase disruption increases longevity and protects against stress. Cell 2007;130:247–58.
37. Boy-Marcotte E, Perrot M, Bussereau F, Boucherie H, Jacquet M. Msn2p and Msn4p control a large number of genes induced at the diauxic transition which are repressed by cyclic AMP in *Saccharomyces cerevisiae*. J Bacteriol 1998;180:1044–52.
38. Schmitt AP, McEntee K. Msn2p, a zinc finger DNA-binding protein, is the transcriptional activator of the multistress response in *Saccharomyces cerevisiae*. Proc Natl Acad Sci U S A 1996;93:5777–82.
39. Smith A, Ward MP, Garrett S. Yeast PKA represses Msn2p/Msn4p-dependent gene expression to regulate growth, stress response and glycogen accumulation. EMBO J 1998;17: 3556–64.
40. Roosen J, Engelen K, Marchal K, et al. PKA and Sch9 control a molecular switch important for the proper adaptation to nutrient availability. Mol Microbiol 2005;55:862–80.
41. Liu K, Zhang X, Lester RL, Dickson RC. The sphingolipid long chain base phytosphingosine activates AGC kinases in *Saccharomyces cerevisiae* including Ypk1, Ypk2 and Sch9. J Biol Chem 2005;280:22679–87.
42. Urban J, Soulard A, Huber A, et al. Sch9 is a major target of TORC1 in *Saccharomyces cerevisiae*. Mol Cell 2007;26:663–74.
43. Harris N, MacLean M, Hatzianthis K, Panaretou B, Piper PW. Increasing *Saccharomyces cerevisiae* stress resistance, through the overactivation of the heat shock response resulting from defects in the Hsp90 chaperone, does not extend replicative life span but can be associated with slower chronological ageing of nondividing cells. Mol Genet Genomics 2001;265:258–63.
44. Herker E, Jungwirth H, Lehmann KA, et al. Chronological aging leads to apoptosis in yeast. J Cell Biol 2004;164:501–7.
45. Madeo F, Herker E, Maldener C, et al. A caspase-related protease regulates apoptosis in yeast. Mol Cell 2002;9:911–7.
46. Wissing S, Ludovico P, Herker E, et al. An AIF orthologue regulates apoptosis in yeast. J Cell Biol 2004;166:969–74.
47. Fabrizio P, Gattazzo C, Battistella L, et al. Sir2 blocks extreme life-span extension. Cell 2005;123:655–67.
48. Blander G, Guarente L. The Sir2 family of protein deacetylases. Annu Rev Biochem 2004;73:417–35.

49. Kimura KD, Tissenbaum HA, Liu Y, Ruvkun G. daf-2, an insulin receptor-like gene that regulates longevity and diapause in *Caenorhabditis elegans*. Science 1997;277: 942–6.
50. Morris JZ, Tissenbaum HA, Ruvkun G. A phospatidylinositol-3-OH kinase family member regulating longevity and diapause in Caenorhabditis elegans. Nature 1996;382:536–9.
51. Paradis S, Ailion M, Toker A, Thomas JH, Ruvkun G. A PDK1 homolog is necessary and sufficient to transduce AGE-1 PI3 kinase signals that regulate diapause in *Caenorhabditis elegans*. Genes Dev 1999;13:1438–52.
52. Hsu AL, Murphy CT, Kenyon C. Regulation of aging and age-related disease by DAF-16 and heat-shock factor. Science 2003;300:1142–5.
53. Ogg S, Paradis S, Gottlieb S, et al. The Forkhead transcription factor DAF-16 transduces insulin-like metabolic and longevity signals in *C. elegans*. Nature 1997;389:994–9.
54. Clancy DJ, Gems D, Harshman LG, et al. Extension of life-span by loss of CHICO, a *Drosophila* insulin receptor substrate protein. Science 2001;292:104–6.
55. Tatar M, Kopelman A, Epstein D, Tu MP, Yin CM, Garofalo RS. A mutant *Drosophila* insulin receptor homolog that extends life-span and impairs neuroendocrine function. Science 2001;292:107–10.
56. Yan LJ, Levine RL, Sohal RS. Oxidative damage during aging targets mitochondrial aconitase [published erratum appears in Proc Natl Acad Sci U S A 1998;95:1968]. Proc Natl Acad Sci U S A 1997;94:11168–72.
57. Orr WC, Sohal RS. Extension of life-span by overexpression of superoxide dismutase and catalase in *Drosophila melanogaster*. Science 1994;263:1128–30.
58. Parkes TL, Elia AJ, Dickinson D, Hilliker AJ, Phillips JP, Boulianne GL. Extension of *Drosophila* lifespan by overexpression of human SOD1 in motorneurons. Nat Genet 1998;19:171–4.
59. Sun J, Tower J. FLP recombinase-mediated induction of Cu/Zn-superoxide dismutase transgene expression can extend the life span of adult *Drosophila melanogaster* flies. Mol Cell Biol 1999;19:216–28.
60. Giannakou ME, Goss M, Junger MA, Hafen E, Leevers SJ, Partridge L. Long-lived Drosophila with overexpressed dFOXO in adult fat body. Science 2004;305:361.
61. Hwangbo DS, Gersham B, Tu MP, Palmer M, Tatar *M. Drosophila* dFOXO controls lifespan and regulates insulin signalling in brain and fat body. Nature 2004;429:562–6.
62. Brown-Borg HM, Borg KE, Meliska CJ, Bartke A. Dwarf mice and the ageing process. Nature 1996;384:33.
63. Flurkey K, Papaconstantinou J, Harrison DE. The Snell dwarf mutation Pit1(dw) can increase life span in mice. Mech Ageing Dev 2002;123:121–30.
64. Coschigano KT, Clemmons D, Bellush LL, Kopchick JJ. Assessment of growth parameters and life span of GHR/BP gene-disrupted mice. Endocrinology 2000;141:2608–13.
65. Holzenberger M, Dupont J, Ducos B, et al. IGF-I receptor regulates lifespan and resistance to oxidative stress in mice. Nature 2003;421:182–7.
66. Bluher M, Kahn BB, Kahn CR. Extended longevity in mice lacking the insulin receptor in adipose tissue. Science 2003;299:572–4.
67. Brown-Borg HM, Rakoczy SG. Catalase expression in delayed and premature aging mouse models. Exp Gerontol 2000;35:199–212.
68. Brown-Borg HM, Rakoczy SG, Romanick MA, Kennedy MA. Effects of growth hormone and insulin-like growth factor-1 on hepatocyte antioxidative enzymes. Exp Biol Med 2002;227:94–104.
69. Kops GJ, Dansen TB, Polderman PE, et al. Forkhead transcription factor FOXO3a protects quiescent cells from oxidative stress. Nature 2002;419:316–21.
70. Rogina B, Helfand SL. Sir2 mediates longevity in the fly through a pathway related to calorie restriction. Proc Natl Acad Sci U S A 2004;101:15998–6003.
71. Tissenbaum HA, Guarente L. Increased dosage of a sir-2 gene extends lifespan in *Caenorhabditis elegans*. Nature 2001;410:227–30.

72. Wood JG, Rogina B, Lavu S, et al. Sirtuin activators mimic caloric restriction and delay ageing in metazoans. Nature 2004;430:686–9.
73. Berdichevsky A, Viswanathan M, Horvitz HR, Guarente L. *C. elegans* SIR-2.1 interacts with 14-3-3 proteins to activate DAF-16 and extend life span. Cell 2006;125:1165–77.
74. Deng H-X, Hentati A, Tainer JH, et al. Amyotrophic lateral sclerosis and structural defects in Cu,Zn superoxide dismutase. Science 1993;261:1047–51.

# Part II
# *Caenorhabditis elegans*

# Chapter 2
# Common Aging Mechanisms: Energy Metabolism and Longevity in *Caenorhabditis elegans*

**Marta Artal-Sanz and Nektarios Tavernarakis**

**Abstract** Aging studies in diverse species ranging from yeast to man have culminated in the delineation of several common signaling pathways that influence the process of senescent decline and aging. Although understanding these interlinked signal transduction cascades is becoming ever more detailed and comprehensive, the cellular and biochemical processes they impinge upon to modulate the rate of senescent decline and aging have lagged considerably behind. This fundamental question is one of the most important challenges of modern aging research and has been the focus of recent research efforts. Emerging findings provide insight into the facets of cellular metabolism that can be fine-tuned by upstream signaling events to ultimately promote longevity. We survey the mechanisms regulating aging in the simple nematode worm *Caenorhabditis elegans*, highlighting recent discoveries that shed light on the interface between aging signaling pathways and cellular energy metabolism. Our objective is to review the current understanding of the processes involved and discuss mechanisms that are likely conserved in higher organisms.

**Keywords** Aging • adipose tissue • *caenorhabditis elegans* • caloric restriction • dauer larva • germline • hormone • insulin • life span • longevity • mitochondrion • reproduction

---

M. Artal-Sanz
Institute of Molecular Biology and Biotechnology, Foundation for Research and Technology, Heraklion, Crete, Greece

N. Tavernarakis (✉)
Institute of Molecular Biology and Biotechnology, Foundation for Research and Technology-Hellas, N. Plastira 100, Vassilika Vouton, P.O. Box 1385, Heraklion GR 70013, Crete, Greece
e-mail: tavernarakis@imbb.forth.gr

C. Sell et al. (eds.), *Life-Span Extension,* Aging Medicine,
DOI 10.1007/978-1-60327-507-1_2,

**Abbreviations** AMP: Adenosine monophosphate; AMPK: AMP-activated protein kinase; ASI: Amphid sensilla I; CR: Caloric restriction; Daf: Dauer larva formation; ETC: Electron transport chain; FOXO: Forkhead; IGF-I: Insulin-like growth factor 1; IIS: Insulin/IGF-I signaling pathway; ILP: Insulin-like peptide; JNK-1: c-Jun N-terminal kinase; L1–L4: Four *Caenorhabditis elegans* larval stages; MST: Mammalian sterile 20-like; PI3K: Phosphatidylinositol 3-kinase; PtdIns: Phosphoinositides; PTEN: Phosphatase and tensin homolog; RNAi: RNA Interference; ROS: Reactive oxygen species.

## 2.1 Introduction

Simple model organisms such as *Caenorhabditis elegans*, *Drosophila melanogaster,* and *Saccharomyces cerevisiae* have provided significant insights that have led to remarkable progress in understanding the molecular pathways that modulate aging and senescence ***(1–4)***. The free-living soil nematode *C. elegans* has been the subject of pioneering research on the genetic regulation of aging in part because of its relatively short life span and its capacity for self-fertilization, which facilitates the generation of genetically homogeneous populations. A multitude of single-gene mutations altering life span have been identified in *C. elegans* and other species, providing evidence that aging can be modulated by evolutionarily conserved regulatory pathways ***(4)***. These pathways normally control growth, reproduction, stress response, and energy metabolism.

In the nematode, neuroendocrine signaling, nutritional sensing, and mitochondrial functions have been shown to play important roles in the determination of life span. We focus on the role of insulin signaling in aging and the mechanisms by which insulin signals are translated through downstream effector kinases and transcriptional factors to modulate life span. In addition, we discuss physiological conditions that affect aging, including dietary restriction, altered mitochondrial function, and reduced protein translation, aiming to highlight links between different pathways that reveal an integrated network of interactions that coordinates the aging process.

## 2.2 The Insulin Signaling Pathway

Aging in *C. elegans* is mainly controlled by the insulin/insulin-like growth factor 1 (IGF-I) signaling pathway (IIS). This neuroendocrine system also modulates life span in flies and mammals, indicating that this pathway is a universal longevity regulator ***(5–7)***. The *C. elegans* IIS pathway was first genetically identified by its effects on the dauer larva formation (Daf) process. Dauer is an alternative nematode developmental stage induced by harsh environmental conditions such as starvation, high population density, or high temperature. Under normal conditions *C. elegans* develops to the reproductive adult through four larval stages (L1–L4) in 3 days.

However, when conditions are adverse, larvae arrest development at the second molt to enter the dauer stage. Dauers do not feed, are resistant to stress, and can survive up to several months. Dauer larvae are considered to be nonaging because postdauer life span is not affected by the duration of the dauer stage ***(8)***. The IIS pathway is central to reproductive growth and metabolism as well as to normal life span. In addition to insulin signaling, the transforming growth factor-β-like pathway also regulates the choice between reproductive growth and dauer entry ***(9)*** and has recently been implicated in the aging process ***(10)***.

The IIS pathway was for the first time linked to aging in *C. elegans* when mutations in two genes, *age-1* and *daf-2* encoding components of the pathway, were found to dramatically extend the life span of the worm ***(6)***. Numerous subsequent investigations have led to the discovery of many additional genes affecting longevity via the IIS pathway.

How does the IIS pathway coordinate physiological processes to influence the aging rate? *C. elegans* senses environmental cues through ciliated sensory neurons. The *C. elegans* genome contains 38 insulin-like ligands that might mediate input to the DAF-2 insulin receptor in response to environmental cues, such as nutritional status or growth conditions ***(11–13)***. Insulin-like peptides (ILPs) can act either as agonists or antagonists on DAF-2 to regulate metabolism, reproductive growth, and life span. ILPs are mainly expressed in neurons, although they are also found in intestine, epidermis, muscle, and gonad. A likely mechanism for the neuroendocrine control of aging is that environmental cues control the production and release of ILPs from sensory cells, thereby influencing the physiology of the organism. Microsurgery or mutations abrogating sensory neurons extend the life span of *C. elegans* ***(14, 15)***. Thus, it is plausible that sensory perception affects life span, at least in part, by influencing the activity of the insulin signaling pathway. However, these manipulations appear to have complicated interactions with the IIS pathway ***(14)***.

DAF-2 is the single *C. elegans* transmembrane insulin receptor kinase ***(16)***. Upon binding of ILPs to DAF-2, the kinase domain of the receptor phosphorylates and activates AGE-1, a phosphatidylinositol 3-kinase (PI3K) ***(17)***. Activated AGE-1 PI3K generates 3-phosphoinositides (PtdIns-3,4-P2 and PtdIns-3,4,5-P3), which are second messengers, required for activation of downstream effector kinases. Downstream kinases include PDK-1, SGK-1, AKT-1, and AKT-2 protein kinase B proteins ***(18–20)***. These protein kinases regulate the forkhead (FOXO) transcription factor DAF-16, which translocates to the nucleus depending on its phosphorylation level ***(21–23)***. Phosphorylated DAF-16 remains inactive in the cytoplasm, whereas upon dephosphorylation it enters the nucleus and exerts its effects on transcription. Thus, the insulin signaling pathway functions to block the nuclear localization of DAF-16. An antagonist of the DAF-2/AGE-1 signaling pathway is the DAF-18/TEN lipid phosphatase ***(24)***. Reduced insulin/IGF-I signaling, increased DAF-18/PTEN (phosphatase and tensin homolog) activity, or stress conditions such as starvation, heat, or oxidative stress result in the nuclear localization of DAF-16/FOXO. In the nucleus, DAF-16 regulates expression of many genes: among others, genes involved in metabolism, immune defense, autophagy, and stress resistance ***(25–28)***.

In addition to the IIS kinase cascade, other kinases modulate DAF-16 activity. The c-Jun N-terminal kinase (JNK-1), a member of the mitogen-activated protein kinase superfamily, is activated by environmental stress, and its overexpression in *C. elegans* results in life extension ***(29)***. JNK-1-mediated life-span extension is DAF-16-dependent. JNK-1 phosphorylates DAF-16 and induces its translocation into the nucleus. JNK-1 overexpression results in increased resistance to oxidative and thermal stress and further increases the life span of *daf-2* mutants. This result indicates that this kinase pathway acts in parallel to the PI3/AKT pathway. The mammalian sterile 20-like (MST) kinase also phosphorylates DAF-16 to regulate oxidative-stress responses and life span ***(30)***. MST is required for mutant *daf-2* longevity, and its overexpression extends life span in a DAF-16-dependent manner. The adenosine monophosphate (AMP)-activated protein kinase (AMPK) senses AMP/ATP ratios and is activated by reduced energy levels. Knockout of the *C. elegans* homologue AAK-2 suppresses mutant *daf-2* longevity whereas its overexpression extends life span ***(31)***. Recent observations indicate that AAK-2 mediates, together with DAF-16, the life-span extension conferred by a specific form of dietary restriction ***(32)***. The authors found that AMPK activates DAF-16-dependent transcription and that it phosphorylates DAF-1/FOXO in vitro at previously unidentified sites ***(32)***. Other kinases partially required for mutant *daf-2* longevity are the p38 MAP kinase and RAS signaling kinases ***(33, 34)***. Apart from phosphorylation, DAF-16/FOXO is also modulated by ubiquitination. The conserved E3 ubiquitin ligase RLE-1 regulates aging by polyubiquitination of DAF-16. RLE-1-deficient worms have increased levels of DAF-16, are stress resistant, and show a *daf-16*-dependent life extension ***(35)***.

Additional factors also regulate DAF-16/FOXO activity in the nucleus. Increased expression of the NAD$^+$-dependent protein deacetylase, sirtuin, increases the life span of yeast, worms, and flies ***(36–38)***. Deacetylation of FOXO by the mammalian homologue SIRT1 is a requirement for its nuclear localization ***(39)***. In *C. elegans*, life span extension conferred by extra copies of *sir-2.1* depends on DAF-16 and on 14–3–3 scaffold proteins. In response to stress, SIRT-2.1, 14–3–3, and DAF-16 form a complex that activates the DAF-16 target gene superoxide dismutase (*sod-3)* ***(40, 41)***. Furthermore, the heat-shock transcription factor HSF-1, which is induced upon heat stress, mediates mutant *daf-2* longevity. HSF-1 overexpression extends life span in a DAF-16-dependent manner ***(42, 43)***. In addition, SMK-1, a conserved nuclear factor, mediates longevity and DAF-16 nuclear localization in worms lacking the germline ***(44)***. Another transcriptional regulator of DAF-16 in worms and mammals is β-catenin/BAR-1, a component of the Wnt signaling pathway. β-catenin physically interacts with DAF-16 and enhances the expression of *sod-3* ***(45)***. However, it is not known whether BAR-1 is required for the long life of insulin/IGF-I signaling mutants.

DAF-16/FOXO is well established as an important mediator of the effects of the IIS pathway. IIS inhibits DAF-16-/FOXO under favorable conditions, and DAF-16 activity is required for the increased longevity and stress resistance that result from reduced IIS. However, DAF-16 is not the only transcription factor directly regulated by IIS. It was recently shown that IIS directly regulates SKN-1, a transcription factor that induces the expression of antioxidant and detoxifying enzymes ***(46)***. SKN-1 is the worm homologue of Nrf2. The increased activity of Nrf2/SKN-1 had been shown to increase stress resistance and to extend the life span of worms and flies ***(1, 47, 48)***. In *C. elegans,* SKN-1 is expressed in the chemosensory amphid sensilla I (ASI) neurons and intestine. The ASI neurons sense food availability and provide endocrine signals that regulate metabolism; expression of SKN-1 in the ASI neurons, but not in the intestine, is required for the life span extension conferred by dietary restriction ***(1)***. In the intestine and in response to stress, SKN-1 localizes to the nucleus and promotes the expression of protective genes ***(1, 47)***. Tullet and colleagues show that defective IIS results in the accumulation of SKN-1 in intestinal nuclei and the upregulation of SKN-1 target genes ***(46)***. The downstream IIS kinases AKT-1, AKT-2, and SGK-1 phosphorylate SKN-1 at multiple sites, sequestering SKN-1 in the cytoplasm. Mutations in any of the three kinases result in the induction of SKN-1-responsive genes. Inductions of some of these genes require DAF-16 whereas others do not. This situation results in a partial overlap on the gene expression programs of DAF-16 and SKN-1 upon reduction of IIS. SKN-1 is required for the longevity phenotype and the stress resistance of IIS deficient worms. SKN-1 delays aging when expressed transgenically, and a mutant form that constitutively localizes to intestinal nuclei extends life span in a DAF-16-independent manner ***(46)***. The intestine is the major fat storage tissue of the worm; in that environment, IIS coordinates at least two transcriptional networks (SKN-1 and DAF-16) that integrate energy metabolism and stress-responsive pathways in response to environmental conditions.

## 2.3 Caloric Restriction

Caloric restriction (CR), a significant reduction in calorie intake without essential nutrient deprivation, can slow the intrinsic rate of aging in yeast, nematodes, flies, rodents, and probably primates ***(49)***. The fascinating effects of dietary restriction include maintenance of most physiological processes in a youthful state and a delay in the occurrence and/or progression of age-associated disease. Little is actually understood about the mechanism by which reduced caloric intake is translated into longevity. In rodents, the antiaging action of dietary restriction is dependent upon the reduced intake of calories rather than on the reduction of the body fat content or metabolic rate ***(50)***.

If the life-prolonging stimulus is reduced calories, what are the molecules that "sense" this signal and convert it to the many physiological changes in calorie-restricted cells? In yeast, CR is mimicked by limiting media glucose levels or by genetic mutation of components of the cyclic AMP-dependent protein kinase A pathway. CR effects on yeast replicative capacity require the activity of the SIR2 histone deacetylase and of NPT1, a gene required for production of NAD, the oxidized form of nicotinamide adenine dinucleotide. NAD availability plays an important role in signaling and may affect several metabolic processes ***(3)***. In *C. elegans*, mutations in genes regulating feeding (*eat* genes) result in lowered food intake caused by defects in pharyngeal function. The consequent, imposed dietary restriction significantly lengthens animal life span ***(51)***. Dietary restriction in worms can also be achieved by diluting their bacterial food. At optimum levels of dietary restriction, worms typically live 2–50% longer than fully fed animals.

How does CR retard aging? Low-calorie intake is correlated with reduced oxidative damage. Thus, the beneficial effects of dietary restriction on life span may depend on its ability to ameliorate oxidative stress by reducing protein oxidation. In addition, dietary restriction has been associated with elevated protein turnover ***(52)***. A recent study confirms earlier reports that protein synthesis and degradation rates decline with age in liver tissue and that this decline is retarded by CR ***(53)***. These findings indicate that elevation of protein turnover and the consequent maintenance of a healthy protein pool, free of oxidant damage, are life span-extending capacities of CR. The molecules that mediate this regulation are of clear interest for antiaging interventions.

Recent research in *C. elegans* has revealed that two evolutionarily conserved transcription factors (PHA-4 and SKN-1) are required for life span extension under dietary restriction ***(1, 54)***. These regulators may coordinate physiological responses to dietary restriction. PHA-4, which was originally described for its role in specifying the pharynx in worm embryos, is a member of the FOXO family of transcription factors and is similar to mammalian FOXA proteins. In mammals, FOXA proteins have developmental roles and regulate glucose metabolism later in life. *pha-4* mutant animals do not respond to dietary restriction. By contrast, mutants lacking DAF-16/FOXO still showed a normal response to dietary restriction, indicating that longevity induced by restricted food intake is DAF-16/FOXO independent. Thus, PHA-4/FOXA appears to be specific for dietary restriction-mediated longevity, whereas DAF-16/FOXO is involved in regulating longevity induced by insulin/IGF-I signaling. A conserved nuclear factor SMK-1 is required for longevity in both pathways ***(54)***.

SKN-1 is related to mammalian NRF2 transcription factors. Similarly to PHA-4, the nematode SKN-1 functions early in embryonic development, where it specifies the formation of the intestine and related tissues. Lack of SKN-1 specifically abolishes dietary-restriction-induced longevity over a wide range of food concentrations without affecting life-span extension through reduction of insulin/IGF signaling ***(1)***. The *skn-1* gene is expressed in the intestine and in a single pair of neurons known as the ASIs. SKN-1 function in the ASI neurons, and not in the intestine, is required for the effects of dietary restriction longevity. Moreover, dietary restriction increases *skn-1* expression specifically in these two neurons. Therefore, dietary restriction activates a highly regulated process rather than passive metabolic changes. Interestingly, ASIs are sensory cells that integrate cues from the environment and produce various hormonal signals that are relayed to the whole body. It is tempting to speculate that these signals coordinate organism-wide physiological responses to dietary restriction.

## 2.4 Mitochondrial Dynamics

Mitochondria are involved in key aging-associated processes such as cellular metabolism, ATP synthesis, and the production and detoxification of reactive oxygen species (ROS). It is, therefore, not surprising that mitochondrial dysfunctions influence the rate of aging. Paradoxically, however, unpaired mitochondrial function often results in increased life span. The first identified mitochondrial long-lived mutant carried lesions in the nuclear gene *clk*-1 ***(55)***, which encodes a mitochondrial protein involved in ubiquinone biosynthesis. Thereafter, a mutation in the *isp-1* gene, encoding the Rieske iron–sulfur subunit of complex III of the electron transport chain (ETC), was also found to increase life span ***(56)***. Other genetic mutations in mitochondrial proteins increasing life span include *gro-1* and *lrs-2*, an isopentenylphosphat/tRNA transferase and a leucine tRNA synthase, respectively ***(11, 57)***. Loss-of-function mutations in ETC components, such as *nuo-1*, *atp-2,* and *frh-1,* increase nematode life span and cause developmental arrest at the L3 larval stage ***(58, 59)***. A genetic mutation in *tpk-1*, a thiamine pyrophosphokinase that affects TCA cycle components, also increases life span ***(60)***. Genome-wide RNA interference (RNAi) screens have identified many other mitochondrial genes, whose reduction results in increased life span. These genes include primarily components of the ETC and ATP synthase, TCA cycle enzymes, and mitochondrial carrier proteins ***(25, 61–64)***.

What is the mechanism by which altered mitochondrial function translates into increased life span? Mitochondria are major producers of ROS because of electron misplacement along the ETC. The free radical theory of aging postulates that ROS cause aging by damaging DNA, lipids, and proteins. In view of this theory, one possibility is that mitochondrial mutations might result in reduced rate of living and decreased ROS production ***(56)***. In other cases, ETC dysfunction might result in increased electron leakage and ROS production, which will consequently activate an adaptive hormetic response and ultimately be beneficial for longevity. That is, in response to mild stress, defense mechanisms will be activated resulting in increased oxidative stress resistance and life extension ***(65, 66)***. Although a handful of data support the oxidative damage theory of aging, recent data put the correlation between oxidative stress and aging into question. Life-extending mitochondrial RNAi interventions respond differently to oxidative stress challenges ***(25, 67)***, indicating lack of correlation between protein oxidation levels and life extension in mitochondrial mutants ***(68)***. Moreover, a measurable increase in oxidative damage due to reduced detoxification does not shorten the life span of long-lived mitochondrial mutants ***(69)***.

Another feasible mechanism involved in life span extension is cellular signaling and the activation of alternative metabolic routes that counter the mitochondrial defect and the energy deficit. Long-lived yeast mitochondrial mutants activate a retrograde signaling pathway that results in the activation of specific transcription factors that will shift metabolism away from the Krebs cycle toward the glyoxylate cycle. This metabolic shift has also been observed in dauer larvae and long-lived *daf-2* mutants ***(70, 71)***. It is possible that a metabolic shift also contributes to the extended life span of *C. elegans* mitochondrial mutants. Reduced AMP/ATP ratios activate AMPK. The *C. elegans* aak-2/AMPK is partially required for the life extension of *daf-2* and mitochondrial mutants ***(31, 72)***. In addition, disruption of *aak-2* abolishes the life-span extension conferred by impaired glycolysis ***(66)***. Recent investigations suggest that cell cycle checkpoint control plays an important role in specifying longevity of mitochondrial mutants ***(68)***.

Many mitochondrial dysfunctions seem to exert their effect on life span independently of the IIS pathway, because, according to some reports, they extend life span independently of DAF-16 and show a synergistic effect with *daf-2* mutations ***(25, 55, 56, 62)***. However, some mitochondrial mutations require DAF-16 for life-span extension and influence its nuclear localization ***(25, 61)***. IIS is coupled to mechanisms that regulate metabolism and oxidative stress. For example, mitochondrial defects are associated with insulin resistance and diabetes. Therefore, it is possible that alteration of mitochondrial function affects longevity, in part, through components of the IIS pathway. To date, no clear mechanistic explanation exists for the observed increased longevity of mitochondrial mutants. Mitochondrial mutations result in pleiotrophic effects and, possibly, different mutations will affect the aging rate differently and in a tissue-specific manner. Certainly, mitochondrial dysfunction results in more intricate physiological responses than merely increasing or reducing oxidative damage. Unveiling the mechanisms implicated in mitochondrial-mediated life extension is crucial to understanding how life span is regulated.

## 2.5 Conclusions

Despite its apparent simplicity, *C. elegans* has a surprisingly sophisticated neuroendocrine system that regulates development, metabolism, and life span. The nervous system performs the task of sensing and integrating environmental cues into coordinated physiological responses that ensure maximal survival and reproductive fitness. In *C. elegans*, food availability, temperature, and a secreted pheromone are some of the sensory inputs that regulate the decision of entering the metabolically active reproductive mode or shifting to the nonreproducing, nonfeeding dauer larva, with large amounts of stored fat. Importantly, the regulation of life span by insulin/IGF-I signaling is conserved across taxa, and reduction of insulin signaling has been shown to extend life span in worms, flies, and mammals. Similarly, the physiological processes involved in the aging process also appear to be conserved. For example, signals from the reproductive system also influence life span in mammals, and dietary restriction has been shown to extend life span in a wide variety of organisms. Likewise, sensory perception could also regulate life span in higher organisms, because blocking the sense of taste reduces insulin secretion in mammals and the smell of food increases insulin levels in humans.

How physiological processes are coordinated by neuroendocrine signaling to meet the biological demands of an organism is still not completely understood. Protein synthesis has emerged as one candidate target process for insulin signaling. Life-span extension caused by decreasing mRNA translation establishes a direct link between protein synthesis and aging. The biological relevance of this relationship is underscored by the tight integration between the IIS pathway and the CR response with mechanisms governing mRNA translation regulation ***(73–75)***. Thus, the effects of insulin/IGF-I signaling and CR on aging could in part be mediated by appropriately modulating protein synthesis, among other processes, to promote longevity.

It is of fundamental importance to understand which cells or tissues emit or receive signals to coordinate the aging process at the level of the whole organism. *C. elegans* has been instrumental for the discovery of conserved molecular pathways regulating aging. Its relatively short life span and its amenability for genetic and molecular analysis make it an ideal organism in which to pursue these studies further, aiming to ultimately understand why and how animals age.

## References


1. Bishop NA, Guarente L. Two neurons mediate diet-restriction-induced longevity in *C. elegans*. Nature 2007;447:545–9.
2. Giannakou ME, Partridge L. Role of insulin-like signalling in Drosophila lifespan. Trends Biochem Sci 2007;32:180–8.
3. Guarente L, Kenyon C. Genetic pathways that regulate ageing in model organisms. Nature 2000;408:255–62.
4. Kenyon C. The plasticity of aging: insights from long-lived mutants. Cell 2005;120:449–60.
5. Bluher M, Kahn BB, Kahn CR. Extended longevity in mice lacking the insulin receptor in adipose tissue. Science 2003;299:572–4.
6. Kenyon C, Chang J, Gensch E, Rudner A, Tabtiang R. A *C. elegans* mutant that lives twice as long as wild type. Nature 1993;366:461–4.
7. Tatar M, Kopelman A, Epstein D, Tu MP, Yin CM, Garofalo RS. A mutant Drosophila insulin receptor homolog that extends life-span and impairs neuroendocrine function. Science 2001; 292:107–10.
8. Klass M, Hirsh D. Non-ageing developmental variant of *Caenorhabditis elegans*. Nature 1976;260:523–5.
9. Ren P, Lim CS, Johnsen R, Albert PS, Pilgrim D, Riddle DL. Control of *C. elegans* larval development by neuronal expression of a TGF-beta homolog. Science 1996;274:1389–91.
10. Shaw WM, Luo S, Landis J, Ashraf J, Murphy CT. The *C. elegans* TGF-beta Dauer pathway regulates longevity via insulin signaling. Curr Biol 2007;17:1635–45.
11. Li W, Kennedy SG, Ruvkun G. *daf-28* encodes a *C. elegans* insulin superfamily member that is regulated by environmental cues and acts in the DAF-2 signaling pathway. Genes Dev 2003; 17:844–58.
12. Pierce SB, Costa M, Wisotzkey R, et al. Regulation of DAF-2 receptor signaling by human insulin and ins-1, a member of the unusually large and diverse *C. elegans* insulin gene family. Genes Dev 2001;15:672–86.
13. Hua QX, Nakagawa SH, Wilken J, et al. A divergent INS protein in *Caenorhabditis elegans* structurally resembles human insulin and activates the human insulin receptor. Genes Dev 2003;17:826–31.
14. Alcedo J, Kenyon C. Regulation of *C. elegans* longevity by specific gustatory and olfactory neurons. Neuron 2004;41:45–5.
15. Apfeld J, Kenyon C. Regulation of lifespan by sensory perception in *Caenorhabditis elegans*. Nature 1999;402:804–9.
16. Kimura KD, Tissenbaum HA, Liu Y, Ruvkun G. *daf-2*, an insulin receptor-like gene that regulates longevity and diapause in *Caenorhabditis elegans*. Science 1997;277:942–6.
17. Morris JZ, Tissenbaum HA, Ruvkun G. A phosphatidylinositol-3-OH kinase family member regulating longevity and diapause in *Caenorhabditis elegans*. Nature 1996;382:536–9.
18. Hertweck M, Gobel C, Baumeister R. *C. elegans* SGK-1 is the critical component in the Akt/PKB kinase complex to control stress response and life span. Dev Cell 2004;6:577–88.
19. Paradis S, Ailion M, Toker A, Thomas JH, Ruvkun G. A PDK1 homolog is necessary and sufficient to transduce AGE-1 PI3 kinase signals that regulate diapause in *Caenorhabditis elegans*. Genes Dev 1999;13:1438–52.

20. Paradis S, Ruvkun G. *Caenorhabditis elegans* Akt/PKB transduces insulin receptor-like signals from AGE-1 PI3 kinase to the DAF-16 transcription factor. Genes Dev 1998;12:2488–98.
21. Henderson ST, Johnson TE. *daf-16* integrates developmental and environmental inputs to mediate aging in the nematode *Caenorhabditis elegans*. Curr Biol 2001;11:1975–80.
22. Lee RY, Hench J, Ruvkun G. Regulation of *C. elegans* DAF-16 and its human ortholog FKHRL1 by the *daf-2* insulin-like signaling pathway. Curr Biol 2001;11:1950–7.
23. Lin K, Hsin H, Libina N, Kenyon C. Regulation of the *Caenorhabditis elegans* longevity protein DAF-16 by insulin/IGF-1 and germline signaling. Nat Genet 2001;28:139–45.
24. Ogg S, Ruvkun G. The *C. elegans* PTEN homolog, DAF-18, acts in the insulin receptor-like metabolic signaling pathway. Mol Cell 1998;2:887–93.
25. Lee SS, Lee RY, Fraser AG, Kamath RS, Ahringer J, Ruvkun G. A systematic RNAi screen identifies a critical role for mitochondria in *C. elegans* longevity. Nat Genet 2003;33:40–8.
26. Melendez A, Talloczy Z, Seaman M, Eskelinen EL, Hall DH, Levine B. Autophagy genes are essential for dauer development and life-span extension in *C. elegans*. Science 2003;301:1387–91.
27. Murphy CT, McCarroll SA, Bargmann CI, et al. Genes that act downstream of DAF-16 to influence the lifespan of *Caenorhabditis elegans*. Nature 2003;424:277–83.
28. Oh SW, Mukhopadhyay A, Dixit BL, Raha T, Green MR, Tissenbaum HA. Identification of direct DAF-16 targets controlling longevity, metabolism and diapause by chromatin immunoprecipitation. Nat Genet 2006;38:251–7.
29. Oh SW, Mukhopadhyay A, Svrzikapa N, Jiang F, Davis RJ, Tissenbaum HA. JNK regulates lifespan in *Caenorhabditis elegans* by modulating nuclear translocation of forkhead transcription factor/DAF-16. Proc Natl Acad Sci U S A 2005;102:4494–9.
30. Lehtinen MK, Yuan Z, Boag PR, et al. A conserved MST-FOXO signaling pathway mediates oxidative-stress responses and extends life span. Cell 2006;125:987–1001.
31. Apfeld J, O'Connor G, McDonagh T, DiStefano PS, Curtis R. The AMP-activated protein kinase AAK-2 links energy levels and insulin-like signals to lifespan in *C. elegans*. Genes Dev 2004;18:3004–9.
32. Greer EL, Dowlatshahi D, Banko MR, et al. An AMPK-FOXO pathway mediates longevity induced by a novel method of dietary restriction in *C. elegans*. Curr Biol 2007;17:1646–56.
33. Nanji M, Hopper NA, Gems D. LET-60 RAS modulates effects of insulin/IGF-1 signaling on development and aging in *Caenorhabditis elegans*. Aging Cell 2005;4:235–45.
34. Troemel ER, Chu SW, Reinke V, Lee SS, Ausubel FM, Kim DH. p38 MAPK regulates expression of immune response genes and contributes to longevity in *C. elegans*. PLoS Genet 2006;2:e183.
35. Li W, Gao B, Lee SM, Bennett K, Fang D. RLE-1, an E3 ubiquitin ligase, regulates *C. elegans* aging by catalyzing DAF-16 polyubiquitination. Dev Cell 2007;12:235–46.
36. Kaeberlein M, McVey M, Guarente L. The SIR2/3/4 complex and SIR2 alone promote longevity in *Saccharomyces cerevisiae* by two different mechanisms. Genes Dev 1999;13:2570–80.
37. Rogina B, Helfand SL. Sir2 mediates longevity in the fly through a pathway related to calorie restriction. Proc Natl Acad Sci U S A 2004;101:15998–6003.
38. Tissenbaum HA, Guarente L. Increased dosage of a *sir-2* gene extends lifespan in *Caenorhabditis elegans*. Nature 2001;410:227–30.
39. van der Horst A, Tertoolen LG, de Vries-Smits LM, Frye RA, Medema RH, Burgering BM. FOXO4 is acetylated upon peroxide stress and deacetylated by the longevity protein hSir2(SIRT1). J Biol Chem 2004;279:28873–9.
40. Berdichevsky A, Viswanathan M, Horvitz HR, Guarente L. *C. elegans* SIR-2.1 interacts with 14–3–3 proteins to activate DAF-16 and extend life span. Cell 2006;125:1165–77.
41. Wang Y, Oh SW, Deplancke B, Luo J, Walhout AJ, Tissenbaum HA. *C. elegans* 14–3–3 proteins regulate life span and interact with SIR-2.1 and DAF-16/FOXO. Mech Ageing Dev 2006;127:741–7.
42. Hsu AL, Murphy CT, Kenyon C. Regulation of aging and age-related disease by DAF-16 and heat-shock factor. Science 2003;300:1142–5.
43. Morley JF, Morimoto RI. Regulation of longevity in *Caenorhabditis elegans* by heat shock factor and molecular chaperones. Mol Biol Cell 2004;15:657–64.

44. Wolff S, Ma H, Burch D, Maciel GA, Hunter T, Dillin A. SMK-1, an essential regulator of DAF-16-mediated longevity. Cell 2006;124:1039–53.
45. Essers MA, de Vries-Smits LM, Barker N, Polderman PE, Burgering BM, Korswagen HC. Functional interaction between beta-catenin and FOXO in oxidative stress signaling. Science 2005;308:1181–4.
46. Tullet JM, Hertweck M, An JH, et al. Direct inhibition of the longevity-promoting factor SKN-1 by insulin-like signaling in *C. elegans*. Cell 2008;132:1025–1038.
47. An JH, Blackwell TK. SKN-1 links *C. elegans* mesendodermal specification to a conserved oxidative stress response. Genes Dev 2003;17:1882–93.
48. Sykiotis GP, Bohmann D. Keap1/Nrf2 signaling regulates oxidative stress tolerance and lifespan in Drosophila. Dev Cell 2008;14:76–85.
49. Sohal RS, Weindruch R. Oxidative stress, caloric restriction, and aging. Science 1996; 273:59–63.
50. Masoro EJ. Caloric restriction and aging: an update. Exp Gerontol 2000;35:299–305.
51. Lakowski B, Hekimi S. The genetics of caloric restriction in *Caenorhabditis elegans*. Proc Natl Acad Sci U S A 1998;95:13091–6.
52. Jazwinski SM. Metabolic control and ageing. Trends Genet 2000;16:506–11.
53. Lambert AJ, Merry BJ. Use of primary cultures of rat hepatocytes for the study of ageing and caloric restriction. Exp Gerontol 2000;35:583–94.
54. Panowski SH, Wolff S, Aguilaniu H, Durieux J, Dillin A. PHA-4/Foxa mediates diet-restriction-induced longevity of *C. elegans*. Nature 2007;447:550–5.
55. Wong A, Boutis P, Hekimi S. Mutations in the clk-1 gene of *Caenorhabditis elegans* affect developmental and behavioral timing. Genetics 1995;139:1247–59.
56. Feng J, Bussiere F, Hekimi S. Mitochondrial electron transport is a key determinant of life span in *Caenorhabditis elegans*. Dev Cell 2001;1:633–44.
57. Lemieux J, Lakowski B, Webb A, et al. Regulation of physiological rates in *Caenorhabditis elegans* by a tRNA-modifying enzyme in the mitochondria. Genetics 2001;159:147–57.
58. Tsang WY, Sayles LC, Grad LI, Pilgrim DB, Lemire BD. Mitochondrial respiratory chain deficiency in *Caenorhabditis elegans* results in developmental arrest and increased life span. J Biol Chem 2001;276:32240–6.
59. Ventura N, Rea S, Henderson ST, Condo I, Johnson TE, Testi R. Reduced expression of frataxin extends the lifespan of *Caenorhabditis elegans*. Aging Cell 2005;4:109–12.
60. de Jong L, Meng Y, Dent J, Hekimi S. Thiamine pyrophosphate biosynthesis and transport in the nematode *Caenorhabditis elegans*. Genetics 2004;168:845–54.
61. Curran SP, Ruvkun G. Lifespan regulation by evolutionarily conserved genes essential for viability. PLoS Genet 2007;3:e56.
62. Dillin A, Hsu AL, Arantes-Oliveira N, et al. Rates of behavior and aging specified by mitochondrial function during development. Science 2002;298:2398–401.
63. Hamilton B, Dong Y, Shindo M, et al. A systematic RNAi screen for longevity genes in *C. elegans*. Genes Dev 2005;19:1544–55.
64. Hansen M, Hsu AL, Dillin A, Kenyon C. New genes tied to endocrine, metabolic, and dietary regulation of lifespan from a *Caenorhabditis elegans* genomic RNAi screen. PLoS Genet 2005;1:119–28.
65. Ventura N, Rea SL, Testi R. Long-lived *C. elegans* mitochondrial mutants as a model for human mitochondrial-associated diseases. Exp Gerontol 2006;41:974–91.
66. Schulz TJ, Zarse K, Voigt A, Urban N, Birringer M, Ristow M. Glucose restriction extends *Caenorhabditis elegans* life span by inducing mitochondrial respiration and increasing oxidative stress. Cell Metab 2007;6:280–93.
67. Kim Y, Sun H. Functional genomic approach to identify novel genes involved in the regulation of oxidative stress resistance and animal lifespan. Aging Cell 2007;6:489–503.
68. Rea SL, Ventura N, Johnson TE. Relationship between mitochondrial electron transport chain dysfunction, development, and life extension in *Caenorhabditis elegans*. PLoS Biol 2007;5:e259.

69. Yang W, Li J, Hekimi S. A measurable increase in oxidative damage due to reduction in superoxide detoxification fails to shorten the life span of long-lived mitochondrial mutants of *Caenorhabditis elegans*. Genetics 2007;177:2063–74.
70. Ruzanov P, Riddle DL, Marra MA, McKay SJ, Jones SM. Genes that may modulate longevity in *C. elegans* in both dauer larvae and long-lived daf-2 adults. Exp Gerontol 2007;42:825–39.
71. Vanfleteren JR, Braeckman BP. Mechanisms of life span determination in *Caenorhabditis elegans*. Neurobiol Aging 1999;20:487–502.
72. Curtis R, O'Connor G, DiStefano PS. Aging networks in *Caenorhabditis elegans*: AMP-activated protein kinase (*aak-2*) links multiple aging and metabolism pathways. Aging Cell 2006;5:119–26.
73. Britton JS, Lockwood WK, Li L, Cohen SM, Edgar BA. Drosophila's insulin/PI3-kinase pathway coordinates cellular metabolism with nutritional conditions. Dev Cell 2002;2:239–49.
74. Holz MK, Ballif BA, Gygi SP, Blenis J. mTOR and S6K1 mediate assembly of the translation preinitiation complex through dynamic protein interchange and ordered phosphorylation events. Cell 2005;123:569–80.
75. Long X, Spycher C, Han ZS, Rose AM, Muller F, Avruch J. TOR deficiency in *C. elegans* causes developmental arrest and intestinal atrophy by inhibition of mRNA translation. Curr Biol 2002;12:1448–61.

# Chapter 3
# Conserved Mechanisms of Life-Span Regulation and Extension in *Caenorhabditis elegans*

**Sean P. Curran**

**Abstract** Human aging correlates with stereotypical changes in physical attributes as well as with an increased incidence of many diseases: atherosclerotic heart disease, cancer, neurological disorders, osteoporosis, obesity, and diabetes. Before we can successfully combat such a wide range of debilitating conditions, a more thorough understanding of the molecular determinants of aging is required. The use of *Caenorhabditis elegans* to identify the basis of human aging has facilitated the rapid identification of genes through a combination of genetic and RNA interference screens. These life-span-controlling genes identified in the worm regulate life span in many organisms and have been shown to play roles in endocrine signaling, reproduction, stress adaptation, metabolism, and genomic maintenance.

**Keywords** *Caenorhabditis elegans* • aging • insulin • dietary restriction • mitochondria • RNA interference • postdevelopmental life span • chemical screens

**Abbreviations** DAF-c: Dauer constitutive; DAF-d: Dauer defective; DR: Dietary restriction; ETC: Electron transport chain; FOXO: Forkhead; IGF-I: Insulin-like growth factor I; PI3K: Phosphatidylinositol-3-OH kinase; PTEN: Phosphatase and tensin homolog; RNAi: RNA interference; ROS: Reactive oxygen species; TGF: Transforming growth factor; TOR: Target of rapamycin

S.P. Curran
Department of Molecular Biology, Massachusetts General Hospital, 185 Cambridge Street, CPZN 7250, Boston, MA, 02114, USA
e-mail: curran@molbio.mgh.harvard.edu

C. Sell et al. (eds.), *Life-Span Extension,* Aging Medicine,
DOI 10.1007/978-1-60327-507-1_3,

## 3.1 *Caenorhabditis elegans* as a Discovery Engine

The use of animals with highly developed genetic infrastructure to study aging has facilitated much of our understanding of how this universal process works. The use of the nematode, *C. elegans*, has yielded some of the most significant discoveries toward elucidating the molecular basis of aging ***(1, 2)***. *C. elegans* is an attractive experimental tool for studying aging for several reasons, including ease of maintenance, its short developmental period (egg to reproductive adult in ~3 days), its short life span (2–3 weeks), and its relatively simple body plan, which consists of 959 somatic cells arising from an invariant pattern of cell division and specification ***(3–5)***. These features and others account for the success of this organism in accelerating the fields of aging, programmed cell death, small RNAs, developmental biology, synaptic transmission, and behavior. The *C. elegans* genome is ~100 Mbp and was the first multicellular eukaryote to be fully sequenced ***(6)***. It has approximately 20,000 protein-coding genes (only 1/3 less than the number found in humans) and ~1,000 noncoding RNAs. There are 2,031 strict human–worm orthologs (bidirection best BLAST hit), and about 35% of all *C. elegans* genes are closely related to human genes.

With increased age comes the susceptibility to numerous debilitating diseases. With advances in medical research, many people are living considerably longer, unmasking an increasing trend toward age-related disease. The elderly tend to be more sedentary; this fact, combined with a decreased metabolic rate, makes them more prone to obesity and diabetes. With age comes an increased probability of disorders of the following systems: neural (decreased cognitive functions and memory); gastrointestinal; renal; genitourinary (prostate enlargement, urinary incontinence); endocrine; cardiovascular (hypertension, coronary heart disease, congestive heart failure, arrhythmia); ear and eye (impaired vision and decreased high frequency acuity); reproductive system (menopause in women and hypogonadism in men); respiratory, hematological, and immune (decreased bone marrow production, increased auto antibodies, anemia); and musculoskeletal (decreased bone density and muscle mass).

Surprisingly, the actual cause of aging remains a mystery, although it has become clear that both genetic and environmental influences play direct roles. Understanding the mechanisms underlying the control of the rate of aging of tissues is fundamental to dissecting the cause of these and other diseases. *C. elegans* has been successfully used to study age-associated human diseases (discussed later) because *C. elegans* displays traits that are similar to those observed during human aging ***(7)*** such as sarcopenia, neural degeneration, reproductive fitness, and metabolic disorders ***(8–18)***.

## 3.2 The Major Axes of Life-Span Regulation in *C. elegans*

The first description of a longevity study using *C. elegans* was that of Michael Klass with David Hirsh in 1976. In this study, Klass described the nonaging state of dauer diapause, an alternative developmental stage similar to hibernation, which would be critical in identifying longevity mutants more than a decade later (see "Endocrine signaling") ***(19)***. Worms can survive in the dauer state for months and then return to the reproductive state with no observable consequence, which is remarkable because the average life span of the worm is typically 2–3 weeks.

In 1977, Michael Klass ***(20)*** described two major biological factors that influence life span in the worm. He showed that the life span of the worm could be modulated by temperature and by the concentration of food provided. He concluded the following:

1. Tradeoffs exist between reproductive fitness and longevity.
2. Life span can be extended by dietary restriction (DR).
3. The pigment lipofuscin accumulates in tissues as they age.
4. Longevity has a genetic component (because the progeny of long-lived adults are also long lived).

An enormous body of research has been dedicated to decoding the genetic components of aging. At the same time, it has become increasingly clear that both stochastic and environmental components regulate life span, although the genetic makeup of an organism is paramount to its level of age-associated, age-related fitness.

### *3.2.1 The Genetics of Aging*

The idea that life span is under genetic control was only recently made popular, and most of the evidence that supported this notion was discovered using *C. elegans*. In humans, at least a portion of the factors influencing life span is thought to be inherited genetically. In studies of adopted twin where the siblings were raised in different households, 75% of the variance in mortality was attributable to "unique environmental factors" ***(21, 22)***. Despite these findings, longevity has a strong genetic component. Siblings of centenarians are four times more likely to live past 85 years than those whose sibling died before age 75 ***(23)***, suggesting a genetic predisposition to longevity.

Klass' initial prediction that aging in the worm was under the control of genetic factors was put to the test by Tom Johnson and Bill Wood in the early 1980s ***(24)***. In their study, two related wild-type strains (Bristol and Bergerac) were mated, and their F1 and F2 progeny were studied for life-span phenotypes. They used these strains to demonstrate that outbred progeny exhibit a spectrum of life spans, each of which is heritably transmitted to subsequent generations.

The first long-lived *C. elegans* genetic mutants were described by Klass in 1983 ***(25)***. Few genes were initially identified as longevity regulators, based solely on longevity phenotypes, because life-span assays are experimentally laborious. Instead, most longevity mutants that were previously isolated were first characterized according to their defects in development, reproduction, food intake, movement, and behavior.

Klass performed the first genetic screen for increased life span and identified the first long-lived mutant in any multicellular species (although he did not know it at the time). His screen yielded many long-lived mutants with uncoordinated (Unc) phenotypes, which arise from deficiencies in muscle or nervous system function. Reasonably, he presumed that the increased longevity of such mutants was likely due to a defect in the efficient ingestion of food, giving rise to a state of caloric restriction. Friedman et al. showed that the increased life-span phenotype associated with the first aging mutant strain could segregate as a single mutation and was stably heritable. Tom Johnson later showed that Klass had generated mutants in the gene for AGE-1 ***(26)***, a PI3 kinase that we now know acts downstream of the insulin receptor/DAF-2 to regulate life span. Further characterization of the *age-1* mutant by Tom Johnson, Pamela Larsen, and Jaques Vanfleteren demonstrated that *age-1* mutants have a decreased rate of mortality, increased thermotolerance, and resistance to oxidative stress, in part due to increased superoxide dismutase and catalase activity. The oxidative stress-resistant phenotype was the first indication of a mechanism that would support the free radical theory of aging ***(27–29)***.

Consistent with its role in the aging processes, *age-1* also regulates the aging-resistant dauer state. Work from Don Riddle and Jim Thomas' laboratories identified a large number of mutants that have dauer constitutive (Daf-c) or dauer defective (Daf-d) phenotypes ***(30–33)***. Genetic analysis shows that the *daf* genes constitute multiple parallel signaling pathways that converge to regulate the diapause decision. In a breakthrough paper, Cynthia Kenyon and colleagues found that the *daf-2* (Daf-c) mutant is long lived (surviving twice as long as wild-type animals) and moreover that the *daf-16* (Daf-d) mutant, which can suppress the dauer phenotype of *daf-2* mutants, also suppressed the long-lived phenotype ***(34)***.

The excitement surrounding the idea of the genetic regulation of life span evolved into hysteria when the molecular identity of *daf-2* and *age-1* were shown by Gary Ruvkun's laboratory to be components of the mammalian insulin signaling cascade. *age-1* encodes the mammalian homolog of the phosphatidylinositol-3-OH kinase (PI3K) p110 catalytic subunit ***(35)***, and *daf-2* is homologous to the upstream mammalian insulin and insulin-like growth factor I (IGF-I) receptors ***(36)***.

The cloning and identification of *daf-16* as a member of the FOXO family of transcription factors by the Ruvkun and Kenyon groups rounded out the identification of the insulin-like signaling cascade in the worm, starting with the extracellular initiation of the signal through the insulin receptor and ending with a transcriptional response via the FOXO transcription factor ***(37, 38)***. Since this initial finding, the insulin-like signaling pathway has been shown also to regulate life span in flies and mice ***(39–43)***.

### 3.2.2 Endocrine Signaling

As previously stated, the insulin-like signaling pathway is a part of a global endocrine system and perhaps represents the most well-studied pathway in *C. elegans* that controls reproductive growth and arrest in the dauer diapause stage. The *daf* classes of genes comprise three parallel signaling pathways (Fig. 3.1): the insulin-like

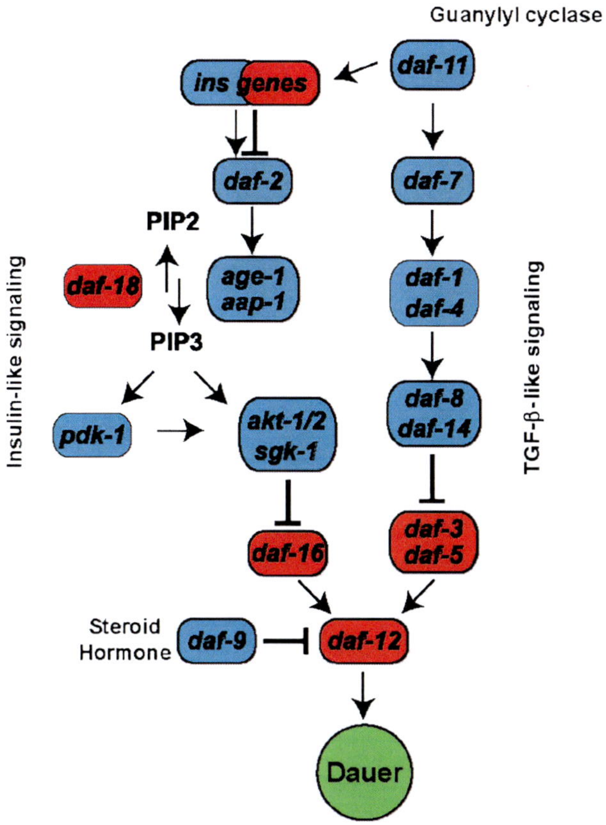


**Fig. 3.1** The *daf* classes of genes comprise three parallel signaling pathways. *TGF-β*, transforming growth factor-β

signaling pathway, the transforming growth factor-β (TGF-β) signaling pathway, and the natriuretic peptide/guanylate cyclase pathway ***(44)***.

### 3.2.2.1 Insulin-Like Signaling

Additional components of the insulin-like signaling cascade have been identified on the basis of mammalian conservation and suppression of the Daf-c phenotype.

*daf-2*, *age-1*, and *pdk-1* are components of the insulin signaling pathway, and partial loss-of-function mutants in this pathway live approximately two to three times longer than wild-type animals ***(27, 34, 36, 45)***. AGE-1/PI3Ks are a class of enzymes that convert $PIP_2$ to $PIP_3$, which binds to the plekstrin homology domain of mammalian AKT/protein kinase B, *akt-1* and *akt-2* in *C. elegans* ***(46, 47)***. The AKTs are phosphorylated by phosphoinositide-dependent kinase-1 (*pdk-1*); *pdk-1* loss-of-function mutation also increases life span by 100% in *C. elegans* ***(46, 48)***.

In addition to the increased life-span phenotype, insulin signaling mutants also display metabolic defects. These mutants misregulate fat ***(36)*** and have decreased metabolism as measured by $CO_2$ production ***(49)***, though in the adult some insulin mutants appear to have normal metabolism ***(49, 50)***. The enhanced life span, metabolic defects, dauer arrest, and stress-resistance phenotypes associated with *daf-2* and *age-1* mutants can be completely suppressed by mutations in *daf-18* (phosphatase and tensin homolog (PTEN) lipid phosphatase) ***(51)*** and *daf-16* (the worm ortholog of the forkhead [FOXO] transcription factors FOXO1/FKHR, FOXO3a/FKHRL1, and FOXO4/AFX) ***(31)***. DAF-18 activity opposes AGE-1 by converting $PIP_3$ back to $PIP_2$. DAF-16 contains four AKT/PKB phosphorylation sites, which regulate DAF-16 cytoplasmic vs. nuclear localization. The insulin signaling pathway negatively regulates DAF-16 by sequestering it in the cytoplasm (Fig. 3.2). Disruption of this insulin signaling cascade releases this inhibition, allowing DAF-16 to move to the nucleus where it regulates an appropriate transcriptional response, which among other effects acts to increase adult life span ***(52–54)***. As in worms, the human DAF-16 homolog FKHRL1 is regulated by Akt, such that mutation of the Akt sites in FKHRL1 causes nuclear localization in the presence of insulin or IGF-I signaling ***(43, 55–59)***.

Although the precise mechanism by which DAF-16 extends life span is not yet understood, we do know from studies in *C. elegans* that DAF-16 regulates the expression of key metabolic and cellular stress-response genes, including detoxification genes ***(53, 54, 60–62)***. The mammalian FOXO transcription factors have subsequently

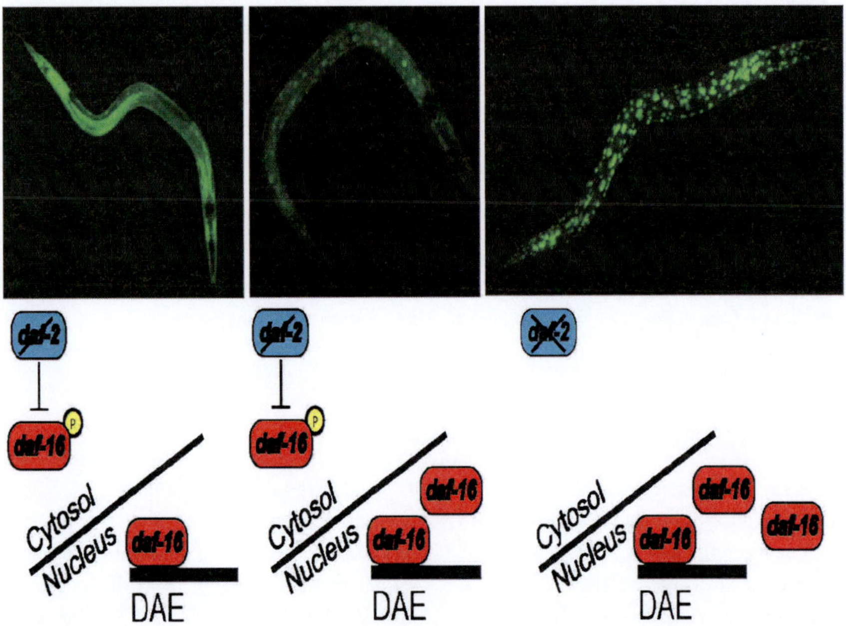


**Fig. 3.2** The insulin signaling pathway negatively regulates DAE-DAF-16 by sequestering it in the cytoplasm

been shown to regulate the expression of these same classes of genes. Human FKHRL1 and *C. elegans* DAF-16 have been shown to bind to the same consensus sequence ***(63–66)***.

Activation of DAF-16 can be accomplished independently of the insulin receptor *daf-2*. Overexpression of the JUN N-terminal kinase *jnk-1* increases life span in a *daf-16*-dependent manner ***(67)***. *jnk-1* is a component of the mitogen-activated protein kinase pathway that, similar to the insulin-like signaling pathway, plays a pivotal role in cellular stress response. Loss-of-function mutations in *lin-14* also result in a *daf-16*-dependent increase in life span ***(68)***. LIN-14 is a novel nuclear protein and potential transcription factor and is a part of a family of heterochronic genes that controls the timing of stage-specific cell lineages and neuronal specificity ***(69–71)***. *lin-14* is a target of the heterochronic microRNA lin-4 ***(72, 73)***. lin-4 functions to downregulate the expression of LIN-14; thus loss of *lin-4* results in increased abundance of LIN-14 and a reduction in life span. Each of these examples requires *daf-16* for the increased life-span phenotype, but both are capable of increasing the life span of hypomorphic insulin signaling mutants.

Mammals are also predicted to use an insulin-like signaling pathway to regulate life span because life span is dramatically increased in dwarf mice with defects in IGF-I signaling and in insulin signaling in fat and neuronal tissues ***(42, 43, 74)***. So why are insulin mutants in the worm long lived whereas defects in insulin signaling in humans cause diabetes? The answer might be as simple as the level of insulin deficiency. All of the mutations in *daf-2* and *age-1* that result in increased life span are hypomorphic. In fact, true null alleles of *daf-2* are lethal and result in embryonic and larval arrest.

#### 3.2.2.2 Transforming Growth Factor-β-Like Signaling

At first, components of the TGF-β-like endocrine pathway (*daf-7*, *daf-1*, *daf-4*, *daf-8*, *daf-14*, *daf-3*) were believed only to regulate dauer diapause and not longevity. *daf-7* codes for the secreted signaling peptide TGF-β ***(75)***, whereas *daf-1* and *daf-4* encode type I and type II TGF-β receptor kinases ***(76, 77)***, respectively. *daf-8* and *daf-14* encode downstream SMAD proteins that function to couple TGF-β signals to the downstream transcriptional regulator DAF-3 ***(78, 79)***. TGB signaling mutants display strong egg-laying (Egl) defects post-dauer decision that causes hatching of eggs in utero, which ultimately kills the parent and disallows life-span assays. Colleen Murphy's laboratory removed this Egl phenotype by chemically sterilizing these mutants with 5-fluoroorоticacid and found that TGF-β pathway mutants were long lived, resembling insulin signaling mutants ***(80)***. Moreover, gene expression analysis revealed that the TGF-β pathway also regulates many of the same genes as the insulin signaling pathway, suggesting that TGF-β and insulin signals may after all function within a single pathway to regulate aging.

Downstream of both TGF-β-like and insulin-like signaling pathways is the steroid hormone receptor, *daf-12*; *daf-12* is homologous to the human vitamin D receptor. At least six phenotypic classes of *daf-12* mutants have been identified.

Some alleles of *daf-12* lead to heterochronic defects. Although most mutants suppress the longevity phenotype of insulin signaling mutants, one class of alleles enhances the increased life-span phenotype of *daf-2* hypomorphic alleles. In the future, studies to characterize the specificities for these two pathways in regulating life span will better clarify the complexities of this endocrine signaling cascade.

#### 3.2.2.3 Tissue Specificity of Endocrine Signaling

Studies to identify the tissues responsible for regulating aging in response to insulin-like signaling in the worm have uncovered some interesting observations. The activity of the insulin receptor and PI3K seems to be most important in neurons, whereas DAF-16 activity is also required in the intestine ***(81, 82)***. This pathway is further complicated by the fact that DAF-16 activity in the intestine regulates DAF-16 activity in other tissues via the insulin-like peptide *ins*-7 ***(83)***.

The *C. elegans* genome codes for 40 insulin-like peptides (*ins* genes), some of which act as DAF-2 (insulin receptor) agonists and others as antagonists ***(84, 85)***. Although it is not well understood why the worm genome codes for so many insulin-like peptides, many members of the *ins* family of genes have risen from recent duplication events and are found in clusters similar to clusters of the insulin superfamily of genes found in humans. Expression analysis of a subset of these insulin-like peptides has shown that they are expressed in various metabolic and neuronal cell types ***(84)***. The *ins-1* gene in the worm is most similar to human insulin.

The Ruvkun laboratory made a transgenic *C. elegans* strain that overexpressed both human and worm *ins-1* and found that both antagonize DAF-2, causing enhanced dauer arrest in wild-type and weak *daf-2* mutants. More importantly, this experiment showed evolutionary conservation at the molecular level of this signaling cascade. Although it was surprising that this agonist peptide (in humans) acted antagonistically (in worms), it could be a result of the cross-species nature of the experiment or of an evolutionary shift in this particular class of insulin-like molecules. The latter maybe true because the *C. elegans ins-1* is also an antagonist.

A separate question is why would insulin-like signaling regulate life span in addition to controlling energetic homeostasis? Are energy utilization and life span connected mechanistically? This mechanism would not have evolved for this strict purpose because postreproductive phenotypes are not under selective pressure but rather as a survival response during harsh and unfavorable conditions. Because endocrine signaling is an essential player in the worm's ability to sense and respond to poor environmental conditions, aspects of this survival response may carry over into adulthood, allowing for effective regulation of life span. The shared use of hormonal control in regulating metabolism and life span suggests that the plasticity of life span across species is due to the release of and response to these hormones; thus, this endocrine network may be ancient in nature ***(86)***.

In mammals, it also appears that the level and location of activity of insulin signaling are the truly important factors. Loss of the insulin receptor in the liver of mice results in a diabetic state, whereas loss of the insulin receptor in adipose tissue makes the animal long lived. In support of the requirement of insulin signaling in neuronal tissues, many gustatory and olfactory neurons have been shown to influence life span in worms and flies, some positively and others negatively ***(87, 88)***. This regulatory system seems to be conserved in humans because the smell of food also increases the level of insulin in humans ***(89)***.

#### 3.2.2.4 *C. elegans* Insulin Signaling and Human Disease

Work from *C. elegans* models for Huntington's disease ***(90)***, sarcopenia ***(8)***, and cancer ***(91)*** has shown that the increase in mean life span resulting from defects in the insulin-like signaling pathway also protects the worm against these age-dependent degenerative conditions.

Humans are much more likely to develop cancer after 60 years of age than those at 30 years of age. Additionally, the probability of being diagnosed with cancer before the 40th year of life is 1:58 for men and 1:52 for women but jumps to 1:11 for men and 1:13 for women between the ages of 40 and 60 and 1:3 for men and 1:4 for women in their 60s and 70s. This phenomenon is evolutionarily conserved because the incidence of cancer in dogs increases at age 10 and in mice at age 1.5. Mutations that stimulate insulin-like signaling also increase the occurrence of cancer (e.g., PTEN tumor suppressor). PTEN mutations activate the cell growth target of rapamycin (TOR) pathway and inhibit the normal downregulation of the FOXO transcription factor that regulates cell growth via p21Cip1 ***(92)*** and apoptosis via fas ligand and bim ***(93, 94)***. Although *C. elegans* does not develop tumors per se, the germ line, which is the only tissue in the worm to remain mitotic in the adult, can overproliferate in response to certain signaling defects. The Kenyon laboratory has recently shown that mutations that increase the life span of worms also act antagonistically with tumor growth. Furthermore, they identified several DAF-16 target genes that regulate tumor growth within the *C. elegans* gonad ***(91, 95)***.

### *3.2.3 Reproduction*

One theory behind the increased longevity found in the insulin-like signaling mutants is that it comes at the expense of reproduction. In some ways this makes sense, because the insulin signaling pathway regulates both reproduction and longevity in *C. elegans* ***(96)***. Some *daf-2* mutants delay reproduction by inducing dauer diapause. These extremely long-lived dauers arrest when the germ line is underdeveloped, perhaps using energy stores for survival and maintenance instead of preparing to produce progeny. From an energetic standpoint, it is conceivable that a decrease in reproductive output could increase the fitness of the organism. In addition, some *daf-2* mutants also delay reproductive senescence, laying eggs well past the normal reproductive period ***(97)***. In studies in human twins, no strong correlation between the age of menarche and menopause has been observed ***(98)***.

Although worm and human reproduction processes are vastly different on many levels, similar to some *daf-2* mutants, human centenarians had a four times greater chance of having a child after the age of 40 than did women who died before the age of 75 ***(23)***.

In an attempt to decouple the reproductive and longevity phenotypes of the insulin-like mutants, Kenyon et al. found that removal of the entire gonad did not affect the life-span increase of *daf-2* mutants ***(34)***, indicating that the signals from the germ line are not required for the longevity observed in *daf-2* mutants. However, in a set of elegant follow-up experiments, the Kenyon laboratory uncovered a complex regulatory system from the germ line.

The *C. elegans* adult hermaphrodite reproductive system stems from four precursor cells named Z1–Z4 ***(5, 34)***. Z1 and Z4 produce the somatic gonad whereas Z2 and Z3 make hundreds of germ cells. In wild-type animals, laser ablation of Z1 and Z4, which removes the entire somatic reproductive system, did not affect life span, as previously shown in *daf-2* mutants. Removal of just the germ cell precursors Z2 and Z3 did, however, result in significant extension similar to that seen with genetic mutants that affect germ-line proliferation, such as *glp-1. glp-1* mutants, which lack germ-line stem cells, display ~60% increase in mean life span ***(99)***. Intriguingly, this life-span extension requires DAF-16, lipophilic-hormone signaling through DAF-12 and *kri-1*, an ankyrin repeat, and FERM domain-containing protein orthologous to human KRIT1 identified by the Kenyon laboratory for DAF-16-dependent life-span extension in germ-line-depleted animals. Notably, KRI-1 functions in the intestine, linking the reproductive and endocrine tissues that regulate life span ***(100)***.

Signaling from the reproductive system also influences life span in mammals. Transferring the ovaries of a young mouse into an old mouse can increase life span by 40–60% ***(101)***. This process kills the endogenous germ cells but leaves the somatic gonad functional. Similarly, a mutation that kills oocytes or low doses of X-irradiation that kills germ cells can increase the life span of flies. Coupling reproduction and aging makes sense from an evolutionary perspective. Mutations that delay reproduction also increase longevity, thus the absolute reproductive period between long-lived and wild-type animals remains the same. Therefore, life span control by signals from the reproductive system is an evolutionarily conserved mechanism and may allow coordination of survival to ensure the passing of genetic material to the next generation.

### *3.2.4 Dietary Restriction*

Since the initial observation by Michael Klass, a significant body of work describes the efforts to understand the mechanism used by DR to extend life span. DR is an evolutionarily conserved regulator of longevity that causes modest increases in life span in yeast, worms, flies, mice, and possibly even humans. Despite its evolutionary conservation, the mechanism underlying this life-span extension is not known.

Characterization of the DR-induced longevity phenotype in the worm has been difficult because too much food can reduce life span and too little food induces starvation and bagging whereby progeny hatch within the parent and mask any potential life-span phenotype ***(102)***. Genetic mutants to mimic the DR phenotype are cleverly named *Eat* mutants and have dysfunctional food-intake rates, which slow feeding. The *Eat* class of mutants is, however, pleiotropic, which potentially confounds the analysis of longevity phenotypes.

Mechanical dilution of the bacterial food source leads to a parabolic effect on life span ***(102)***. Food dilution extends the reproductive period of the worm but also restricts brood size, similar to several insulin-like signaling mutants (discussed earlier). Although the specific mechanism of DR on extending life span is not known, characterization of the *eat* mutants and bacterial dilution DR models has revealed that these pathways may mediate increased life span via increased responsiveness to some stresses. In DR-treated animals, superoxide dismutase and catalase activity are significantly increased, but no increased tolerance to paraquat and thermal stress is observed ***(103)***. To complicate the issue further, the use of axenic media (another form of DR) does result in resistance to paraquat, similar to the oxidative stress-resistance phenotypes of DR mice ***(104)***. Perhaps most amazing is the observation that complete removal of food significantly extends the life span of *C. elegans*, although this dietary regimen will be less appealing to many people ***(105)***. Kaeberlein et al. have shown that starvation can induce strong longevity phenotypes and that this increase in life span is not at the cost of fertility because the same effects can be seen when starvation is induced postreproductively.

So which experiment truly generates a state of DR in the worm? Perhaps they all do. A more detailed characterization of each method will, however, undoubtedly lead to a better understanding of the molecular mechanisms involved. The search for genetic determinants of DR-mediated life-span extension has only led to more questions.

In mammals, DR has been shown to decrease the levels of insulin. In light of this finding, the increase in life span associated with decreased DAF-2 signaling in the worm may be analogous to mammalian longevity increases by caloric restriction ***(106)***. The pancreas secretes insulin in a nutrient-dependent manner that is regulated by autonomic neurons. Insulin binds to the insulin receptor at the plasma membrane of metabolic tissues, triggering the coordinated expression of metabolic enzymes that can break down glucose, amino acids, and fat. Perhaps not surprisingly, life span in *C. elegans* is also tied to feeding rate, which is similar to DR in mammals and flies. Despite these similarities, DR in the worm at first glance appears not to be part of the insulin signaling cascade because it acts independently of the FOXO transcription factor *daf-16* ***(107)***.

The sirtuin (SIR2) proteins are a class of evolutionarily conserved deacetylases that act to extend life span across many species ***(108)***. In flies and yeast, SIR2 is required for DR-induced longevity ***(109, 110)***. In the worm it is unclear if DR requires the worm ortholog *sir-2.1*. In addition, the increased life-span phenotype resulting from *sir-2.1* overexpression requires *daf-16* ***(111)***. Because *daf-16* is not required for DR-induced longevity but is the major target in the insulin-like signaling pathway, it seemed possible that *sir-2.1* is a part of the insulin signaling pathway ***(103)***. However, Wang and Tissenbaum found that *sir-2.1* loss-of-function mutants suppress the longevity phenotype of *eat-2* mutants but not of *daf-2* mutants ***(112)***. Therefore, perhaps *sir-2.1* functions to bridge DR and insulin-like signaling in the worm. In mammals, SirT1 deacetylates FOXO and leads to the increased expression of stress-response genes ***(113, 114)***.

TOR has been implicated in regulating DR in flies and yeast ***(115, 116)***. *tor1* mutants in yeast increase both chronological and replicative aging but do not further increase life span compared with yeast undergoing DR. Similar to *sir-2.1*, TOR (*let-363*) in worms is activated by the insulin-like signaling pathway and DAF-15 (raptor) is repressed by DAF-16 ***(117, 118)***. *daf-16(lf)* mutants do not suppress the extended life-span phenotype of *let-363* inactivation; however, no synergy exists between *let-363* and *daf-2* mutants, suggesting that these pathways are one and the same.

Two genes, *pha-4* and *skn-1*, that specifically regulate the DR longevity phenotype have recently been identified. PHA-4 is the *C. elegans* FoxA transcription factor ortholog and SKN-1 is homologous to the NRF (NF-E2-related factor) family of transcription factors ***(119, 120)***. These genes specifically regulate DR-mediated longevity in the worm. Of additional interest, *skn-1* functions in the ASI neurons in support of a neuroendocrine regulatory circuit of life-span control. The identification of these two genes is a powerful start to understanding the genetic control of life span and will undoubtedly facilitate the discovery of more genetic loci that control aging both specific to DR and to longevity control in general.

### 3.2.5 Mitochondria

In a screen for maternally rescued viable mutations in *C. elegans*, Lakowski and Hekemi identified three Clock (*Clk*) genes and *gro-1*, which exhibit slow development and increased life span ***(121)***. In this study, double mutant analysis with *age-1* placed the *clk* genes in an independent regulatory pathway from the insulin signaling, because the double mutant was significantly longer lived than either single mutant. However, the *age-1* and *clk-1* alleles used are not null mutations; therefore, the increase in life span observed could be the result of adding the phenotypes associated with two hypomorphic mutations.

The molecular identification of *clk-1* ***(122)*** revealed homology to a mitochondrial gene that regulates coenzyme $Q_9$ (Q) biosynthesis (a component of the mitochondrial electron transport chain [ETC]), thus potentially reducing the metabolic output of the animal. *clk-1* mutants require Q derived from *Escherichia coli* for proper development as well as for fertility ***(123, 124)***. The animals lacking endogenous Q but fed a Q-replete *E. coli* food source are long lived. Wild-type worms fed a Q-less diet are long lived, and this life-span extension is independent of *daf-16* and *daf-12* ***(125)***. The *clk-1* mechanism of regulating life span is evolutionarily conserved; mice with a heterozygous mutation in the *clk-1* ortholog display a significantly longer life span than their wild-type littermates ***(126)***.

Genetic screens to phenocopy the Clk phenotype identified another mitochondrial gene involved in iron–sulfur cluster biogenesis, *isp-1* ***(127)***. *isp-1* mutants are long lived, have decreased metabolism as gauged by reduced oxygen consumption, and show directly that mitochondrial electron transport is a key determinant of life span. This pathway is independent of the insulin signaling pathway, because decreased ETC activity can further extend the life span of both long-lived *daf-2* mutants and short-lived *daf-16* mutants ***(128)***.

How does crippling the ETC lead to an increase in life span? The mitochondria, in addition to acting as the powerhouse of the cell, also act as a toxic house, producing a major source of oxidative stress by releasing reactive oxygen species (ROS) into the cytosol. ROS are toxic due to their ability to damage the essential structures of DNA, RNA, and proteins. Balancing ROS production and ATP output by regulating mitochondrial activity could elegantly regulate life span. Not all mitochondrial loss-of-function mutations result in an increased life-span phenotype. *mev-1(kn1)* mutants have higher levels of ROS, decreased respiration, hypersensitivity to paraquat, and decreased life span ***(129)***. *mev-1* codes for the cytochrome *b* large subunit of complex II. The fact that mitochondrial mutations can lead either to an increase or to a decrease in life span is perplexing. One possibility is that reduced respiration in all mitochondrial mutants uniformly acts to increase longevity; however, this increase can be negated by the increased production of ROS in a subset of mitochondrial mutants.

## 3.3 Next Generation Studies to Identify Life-Span Regulators

In the first 30 years of *C. elegans* aging research, ~15 genes were identified that regulate life span. The transition from the twentieth to the twenty-first century brought with it the first genome-wide RNA interference (RNAi) screens in *C. elegans*. The ability to selectively knock down a specific gene and look for a desired phenotype (longevity) revolutionized the aging research community. The strong influence of mitochondria on life span became apparent during the first attempts at large-scale RNAi screens for increased life span, which identified several mitochondrial genes ***(55, 128)***.

### *3.3.1 RNA Interference*

RNA interference in *C. elegans* can be initiated by delivering dsRNA against a specific gene by injection, soaking, or feeding ***(130–132)***. In feeding RNAi, *E. coli* (the laboratory food source of *C. elegans*) is engineered to produce double-stranded RNA corresponding to each of the ~22,000 *C. elegans* genes (Fig. 3.3). In brief, the gene of interest is placed between two T7 promoter sites on opposing strands. Induction of T7 RNA polymerase synthesizes two complementary RNAs, which

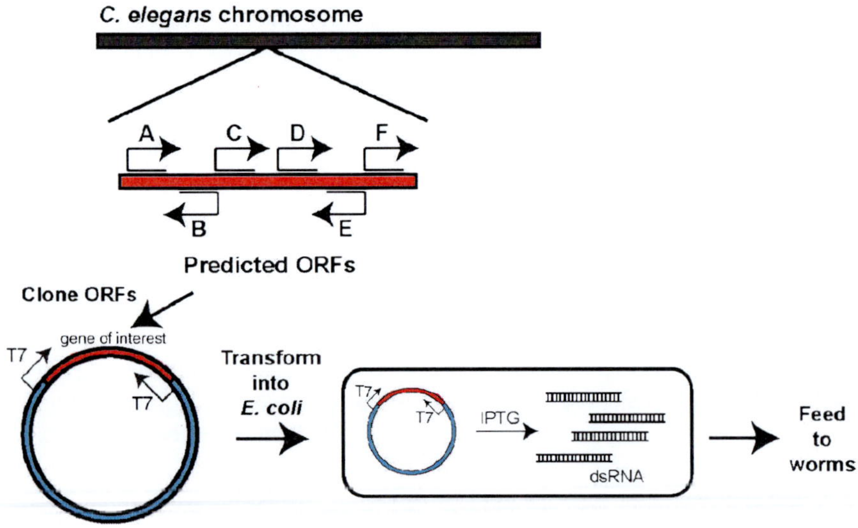


**Fig. 3.3** RNA interference initiated by feeding. *Escherichia coli* (the laboratory food source of *Caenorhabditis elegans*) is engineered to produce double-stranded RNA (dsRNA) corresponding to each of the ~22,000 *C. elegans* genes. IPTG, isopropyl β-D-1-thiogalactopyranoside; ORF, open reading frame

hybridize to create a dsRNA targeting the gene of interest. Feeding each of these clones individually to worms allows for the specific knockdown of each gene in the genome. The Ahringer and Vidal laboratories have created two independent libraries that together cover most of the predicted genes in the *C. elegans* genome, allowing for genome-wide coverage when screening ***(133, 134)***.

#### 3.3.1.1 RNAi Screens for Increased Life-Span Phenotypes

Genome-wide RNAi screens have been used to identify key regulators of life span as well as genes that regulate age-related diseases such as alpha-synuclein inclusion formation ***(135)*** and polyglutamine pathogenesis ***(136)***. Four large-scale RNAi screens have been performed to identify negative regulators of life span ***(55, 137, 138, 140)***.

The first of these screens for increased life span analyzed RNAi clones that targeted most of the genes on chromosome I. This screen of ~5,700 gene inactivations found an enrichment for clones that target mitochondrial function ***(55)***. In a separate screen, RNAi was used to inactivate the nuclear coded genes for the ETC and mitochondrial ATPase ***(139)***. Similar to mitochondrial genetic mutants, RNAi to mitochondrial genes resulted in increased life span.

Two genome-wide RNAi approaches in *C. elegans* identified 118 genes that when knocked down can significantly increase mean life span from 7 to 87% ***(137, 140)***. These screens successfully identified known regulators of life span including components of the insulin signaling pathway and genes that regulate mitochondrial function and metabolism. One additional benefit of using RNAi is the ability to quickly perform "pseudo" epistasis experiments. RNAi clones that induce a specific phenotype in one genetic background can be immediately screened for suppression or enhancement in other distinct genetic backgrounds, provided the mutation is a null allele. The Lee and Kenyon groups rescreened each of their RNAi clones in a *daf-16* null background looking for genes that function in the insulin signaling pathway. Both screens identified a significant number of genes that require the FOXO transcription factor for life-span extension and are likely part of or converge on the insulin signaling pathway. In addition, Hamilton et al. ***(137)*** rescreened their putative longevity regulators in the *sir-2.1* null background. Interestingly, nine of their genes require both *daf-16* and *sir-2.1* for life-span extension and probably act upstream of these two gene products.

The idea that genome-wide RNAi screens are comprehensive and that RNAi itself is a reliable means for gene knockdown has been put to the test ***(141)***. If this observation were true, each of these screens should identify all the known regulators of life span and independently identify the same longevity regulators. The first of these predictions was partially fulfilled by both screens. Both of these screens identified known components of the insulin signaling pathway including *daf-2* ***(140)*** and *age-1* and *akt-1* ***(137)***. These two screens, however, identified mostly nonoverlapping sets of longevity regulators. This result is most likely due to the differences in screening conditions, strain background, and statistical criteria for scoring positive in the screen. It has been shown that feeding RNAi often yields false-negative phenotypes. But why were all known components not identified? This result can partially be explained by the nature of RNAi itself. RNAi-mediated gene inactivation is genetically analogous to hypomorphy. The ability to effectively knock down expression is dependent on a number of factors including but not limited to the amount of dsRNA produced, the amount ingested by the worm and functionally utilized, and the ability of specific cell types to respond to the dsRNA (neurons are particularly refractory to RNAi) ***(132)***. With this in mind, it is likely that these screens are far from saturating and that repeating each screen and/or improving the efficacy of RNAi will identify new regulators of life span.

#### 3.3.1.2 Specialized RNAi Screens for Life-Span Phenotypes

Even with these difficulties, RNAi provides two unique features for reducing gene expression. First, RNAi can be initiated at any time, ranging from the L1 stage throughout development and into adulthood. Adult hermaphrodites can be fed RNAi, and embryos can be screened for developmental defects. Dillin et al. beautifully demonstrated the power of this advantage by analyzing the temporal requirements for life-span extension by inactivating genes in the insulin signaling pathway and ETC ***(139)***. What is perhaps most interesting is the differences in timing of knockdown for these two pathways and the concomitant impact on longevity. RNAi targeting components of the insulin-like signaling pathway can be shut down at any point in development, even in the postreproductive adult, to increase life span. In contrast, components of the ETC must be knocked down during development to receive the life-span benefit, although use of enhanced RNAi mutants does yield some, albeit less dramatic, increase in life span with postdevelopmental exposure to RNAi targeting mitochondrial genes ***(128, 138)***. These results predict that some components of life span are determined early in development whereas others retain their ability to regulate longevity postdevelopmentally. The second strength of RNAi is actually the ability to produce reduced function phenotypes for essential genes. For instance, the null phenotype of the insulin receptor *daf-2* is lethal whereas partial loss-of-function results in increased adult life span. RNAi thus provides the ability to analyze genes whose null phenotype is lethal and would otherwise be difficult to work with.

The theory of antagonistic pleiotropy ***(142)*** suggests that certain genes have an essential role early in development but lead to reduced fitness later in life. Inspired by this theory, the Ruvkun laboratory analyzed this "essential" class of genes ***(138)***. The two initial genome-wide approaches began RNAi treatment from the earliest larval stage and then scored adults for extended longevity. As such, these analyses excluded approximately 2,700 gene inactivations that result in early arrest or lethality prior to adulthood. Significantly, this class of essential genes is much more likely to be conserved in phylogeny than are genes with no developmental phenotype. Because this observation is true, a screen of such genes would have an increased likelihood to enrich for genes with relevance to longevity control in higher animals. With this idea in mind, Curran and Ruvkun devised a pair of screens of essential genes. In the first screen, RNAi feeding was initiated as animals entered adulthood; adult longevity was scored, thus bypassing early essential functions for these genes. In the second screen, L1s were fed RNAi against essential genes, and animals that underwent a developmental arrest were scored for longevity. In support of their hypothesis, they identified 64 essential genes that when inactivated postdevelopmentally yielded potent extension of life span. In fact, despite the inactivation starting at adulthood, some of the RNAi clones induced some of the strongest life-span phenotypes documented. This screen identified known genes that regulate life span via the canonical longevity-promoting pathways in addition to pathways not previously implicated in aging, including enrichment of RNA and chromatin factors and genes involved in protein synthesis.

Concurrent with the Ruvkun study, the Kapahi laboratory conducted an independent screen of 57 essential genes and found that postdevelopmental knockdown of 23 of these genes increased life span ***(143)***. These two screens identified some of the same genes but more importantly enriched for many of the same biological processes. One such process that has arisen as a potent regulator of life span is control of protein synthesis ***(144)***. The decrease in life span as a result of the downregulation of protein synthesis could be attributed to a surplus of energy equivalents that can be redirected to other cellular processes and too a decrease in erroneously synthesized polypeptides, thus freeing cytosolic chaperones and protein turnover machinery to deal with other cellular proteins in need of repair or destruction ***(145)***.

Life-span assays are population based, which makes screening mutagenized animals using standard genetics extremely laborious. Even more complicated is the study of short life span and suppression of long life span. In the first screen to identify genes required to extend life span, the Ruvkun laboratory performed a genome-wide RNAi screen to suppress the long-lived phenotype of *daf-2* mutants ***(146)***. Using detailed secondary assays, gene inactivations that result in general "sickness" and that were not specific to insulin-mediated longevity pathways were ruled out. This screen identified numerous factors, including some previously shown to be responsible for the extended longevity of *daf-2* mutants, such as components of the endocytosis pathway ***(147)***, *smk-1* ***(148)***, and *daf-16* ***(34)***. In similar fashion, future RNAi screens can be performed to identify specific regulators of DR and mitochondrial pathways for regulating life span.

RNAi in *C. elegans* has enabled some of the most comprehensive studies of life span in any model system. As the mechanisms underlying RNAi are more rigorously studied, the utility of this method will undoubtedly provide even more discoveries concerning the molecular basis of aging.

### 3.3.2 Chemical Screens

One of the newest and perhaps most immediately applicable approaches in *C. elegans* and other systems toward facilitating life-span extension in humans is the use of small-molecule screens for life-span phenotypes. Over the last decade, numerous chemicals have been tested on *C. elegans* for induction of life-span phenotypes: superoxide dismutase/catalase mimetics ***(149)***, resveratrol and other sirtuin activators ***(109, 110)***, valproic acid ***(150)***, alpha-tocopherol ***(151)***, anticonvulsant drugs ***(152)***, blueberry polyphenols ***(153)***, and antidepressant drugs ***(154)***.

In the first large-scale chemical screen, Linda Buck's research group analyzed 88,000 chemicals and found 115 that statistically increased life span, 13 of which could increase life span 30–60%. One compound was similar to a human antidepressant that alters serotonin signaling. They then tested additional chemicals known to target serotonin-signaling regulators and identified four additional compounds that similarly affected life span. Screens such as these are particularly exciting because the drugs tested already have Food and Drug Administration approval and could be tested more quickly in mammals for similar effects.

The next step in these studies is to test delivery of these drugs in other model systems and to identify the molecular targets of these compounds. These aims have been successfully accomplished for resveratrol. Resveratrol targets the sirtuin family of deacetylases, and resveratrol has been shown to increase life span in most model organisms ***(109, 110, 155)***.

Although chemical screens have only recently become widely used in the *C.elegans* research community, the immediate impact of such screens will undoubtedly hasten the goals of the researchers using *C. elegans* as a model system to study aging. These compounds may not be immediately applicable for human use, but the *C. elegans* model system will further facilitate identification of the mechanisms utilized by these drugs so that they may be better used to modulate the phenotypes associated with increased age in humans.

**Acknowledgments** Special thanks to members of the Ruvkun laboratory for comments on this chapter and to the NIH for funding. I regret that, due to length limitations, I could not acknowledge all the studies on aging of the *C. elegans* research community.

## References

1. Wolff S, Dillin A. The trifecta of aging in *Caenorhabditis elegans*. Exp Gerontol 2006; 41:894–903.
2. Kenyon C. The plasticity of aging: insights from long-lived mutants. Cell 2005;120:449–60.
3. Brenner S. The genetics of *Caenorhabditis elegans*. Genetics 1974;77:71–94.
4. Sulston JE, Schierenberg E, White JG, Thomson JN. The embryonic cell lineage of the nematode *Caenorhabditis elegans*. Dev Biol 1983;100:64–119.
5. Sulston JE, Horvitz HR. Post-embryonic cell lineages of the nematode, *Caenorhabditis elegans*. Dev Biol 1977;56:110–56.
6. *C. elegance* Sequencing Consortium. Genome sequence of the nematode *C. elegans*: a platform for investigating biology. Science 1998;282:2012–8.
7. Johnson TE. Aging can be genetically dissected into component processes using long-lived lines of *Caenorhabditis elegans*. Proc Natl Acad Sci U S A 1987;84:377–81.
8. Herndon LA, Schmeissner PJ, Dudaronek JM, et al. Stochastic and genetic factors influence tissue-specific decline in ageing *C. elegans*. Nature 2002;419:808–14.
9. Chalfie M. Touch receptor development and function in *Caenorhabditis elegans*. J Neurobiol 1993;24:1433–41.
10. Johnston J, Iser WB, Chow DK, Goldberg IG, Wolkow CA. Quantitative image analysis reveals distinct structural transitions during aging in *Caenorhabditis elegans* tissues. PLoS ONE 2008;3:e2821.
11. Hughes SE, Evason K, Xiong C, Kornfeld K. Genetic and pharmacological factors that influence reproductive aging in nematodes. PLoS Genet 2007;3:e25.
12. Murakami S. *Caenorhabditis elegans* as a model system to study aging of learning and memory. Mol Neurobiol 2007;35:85–94.
13. Ventura N, Rea SL, Testi R. Long-lived *C. elegans* mitochondrial mutants as a model for human mitochondrial-associated diseases. Exp Gerontol 2006;41:974–91.
14. Olsen A, Vantipalli MC, Lithgow GJ. Using *Caenorhabditis elegans* as a model for aging and age-related diseases. Ann N Y Acad Sci 2006;1067:120–8.
15. Bossy-Wetzel E, Barsoum MJ, Godzik A, Schwarzenbacher R, Lipton SA. Mitochondrial fission in apoptosis, neurodegeneration and aging. Curr Opin Cell Biol 2003;15:706–16.
16. Barbieri M, Bonafe M, Franceschi C, Paolisso G. Insulin/IGF-I-signaling pathway: an evolutionarily conserved mechanism of longevity from yeast to humans. Am J Physiol Endocrinol Metab 2003;285:E1064–71.
17. Tsang WY, Lemire BD. The role of mitochondria in the life of the nematode, *Caenorhabditis elegans*. Biochim Biophys Acta 2003;1638:91–105.
18. Wallace DC. Animal models for mitochondrial disease. Methods Mol Biol 2002;197:3–54.
19. Klass M, Hirsh D. Non-ageing developmental variant of *Caenorhabditis elegans*. Nature 1976;260:523–5.
20. Klass MR. Aging in the nematode *Caenorhabditis elegans*: major biological and environmental factors influencing life span. Mech Ageing Dev 1977;6:413–29.
21. Herskind AM, McGue M, Holm NV, Sorensen TI, Harvald B, Vaupel JW. The heritability of human longevity: a population-based study of 2872 Danish twin pairs born 1870–1900. Hum Genet 1996;97:319–23.
22. Ljungquist B, Berg S, Lanke J, McClearn GE, Pedersen NL. The effect of genetic factors for longevity: a comparison of identical and fraternal twins in the Swedish Twin Registry. J Gerontol A Biol Sci Med Sci 1998;53:M441–6.

23. Perls T, Kohler IV, Andersen S, et al. Survival of parents and siblings of supercentenarians. J Gerontol A Biol Sci Med Sci 2007;62:1028–34.
24. Johnson TE, Wood WB. Genetic analysis of life-span in *Caenorhabditis elegans*. Proc Natl Acad Sci U S A 1982;79:6603–7.
25. Klass MR. A method for the isolation of longevity mutants in the nematode *Caenorhabditis elegans* and initial results. Mech Ageing Dev 1983;22:279–86.
26. Friedman DB, Johnson TE. A mutation in the age-1 gene in *Caenorhabditis elegans* lengthens life and reduces hermaphrodite fertility. Genetics 1988;118:75–86.
27. Larsen PL. Aging and resistance to oxidative damage in *Caenorhabditis elegans*. Proc Natl Acad Sci U S A 1993;90:8905–9.
28. Vanfleteren JR. Oxidative stress and ageing in *Caenorhabditis elegans*. Biochem J 1993;292 (Pt 2):605–8.
29. Johnson TE. Increased life-span of age-1 mutants in *Caenorhabditis elegans* and lower Gompertz rate of aging. Science 1990;249:908–12.
30. Golden JW, Riddle DL. The *Caenorhabditis elegans* dauer larva: developmental effects of pheromone, food, and temperature. Dev Biol 1984;102:368–78.
31. Gottlieb S, Ruvkun G. daf-2, daf-16 and daf-23: genetically interacting genes controlling Dauer formation in *Caenorhabditis elegans*. Genetics 1994;137:107–20.
32. Schackwitz WS, Inoue T, Thomas JH. Chemosensory neurons function in parallel to mediate a pheromone response in *C. elegans*. Neuron 1996;17:719–28.
33. Thomas JH, Birnby DA, Vowels JJ. Evidence for parallel processing of sensory information controlling dauer formation in *Caenorhabditis elegans*. Genetics 1993;134:1105–17.
34. Kenyon C, Chang J, Gensch E, Rudner A, Tabtiang R. A *C. elegans* mutant that lives twice as long as wild type. Nature 1993;366:461–4.
35. Morris JZ, Tissenbaum HA, Ruvkun G. A phosphatidylinositol-3-OH kinase family member regulating longevity and diapause in *Caenorhabditis elegans*. Nature 1996;382:536–9.
36. Kimura KD, Tissenbaum HA, Liu Y, Ruvkun G. daf-2, an insulin receptor-like gene that regulates longevity and diapause in *Caenorhabditis elegans*. Science 1997;277:942–6.
37. Ogg S, Paradis S, Gottlieb S, et al. The Fork head transcription factor DAF-16 transduces insulin-like metabolic and longevity signals in *C. elegans*. Nature 1997;389:994–9.
38. Lin K, Dorman JB, Rodan A, Kenyon C. daf-16: An HNF-3/forkhead family member that can function to double the life-span of *Caenorhabditis elegans*. Science 1997;278:1319–22.
39. Clancy DJ, Gems D, Harshman LG, et al. Extension of life-span by loss of CHICO, a Drosophila insulin receptor substrate protein. Science 2001;292:104–6.
40. Tatar M, Kopelman A, Epstein D, Tu MP, Yin CM, Garofalo RS. A mutant Drosophila insulin receptor homolog that extends life-span and impairs neuroendocrine function. Science 2001;292:107–10.
41. Hwangbo DS, Gershman B, Tu MP, Palmer M, Tatar M. Drosophila dFOXO controls lifespan and regulates insulin signalling in brain and fat body. Nature 2004;429:562–6.
42. Holzenberger M, Dupont J, Ducos B, et al. IGF-1 receptor regulates lifespan and resistance to oxidative stress in mice. Nature 2003;421:182–7.
43. Bluher M, Kahn BB, Kahn CR. Extended longevity in mice lacking the insulin receptor in adipose tissue. Science 2003;299:572–4.
44. Hu PJ. Dauer. WormBook 2007:1–19.
45. Dorman JB, Albinder B, Shroyer T, Kenyon C. The age-1 and daf-2 genes function in a common pathway to control the lifespan of *Caenorhabditis elegans*. Genetics 1995;141:1399–406.
46. Paradis S, Ailion M, Toker A, Thomas JH, Ruvkun G. A PDK1 homolog is necessary and sufficient to transduce AGE-1 PI3 kinase signals that regulate diapause in *Caenorhabditis elegans*. Genes Dev 1999;13:1438–52.
47. Alessi DR, Andjelkovic M, Caudwell B, et al. Mechanism of activation of protein kinase B by insulin and IGF-1. EMBO J 1996;15:6541–51.
48. Alessi DR, James SR, Downes CP, et al. Characterization of a 3-phosphoinositide-dependent protein kinase which phosphorylates and activates protein kinase Balpha. Curr Biol 1997;7:261–9.
49. Van Voorhies WA, Ward S. Genetic and environmental conditions that increase longevity in *Caenorhabditis elegans* decrease metabolic rate. Proc Natl Acad Sci U S A 1999;96:11399–403.

50. Gems D. Nematode ageing: putting metabolic theories to the test. Curr Biol 1999;9:R614–6.
51. Ogg S, Ruvkun G. The *C. elegans* PTEN homolog, DAF-18, acts in the insulin receptor-like metabolic signaling pathway. Mol Cell 1998;2:887–93.
52. Oh SW, Mukhopadhyay A, Dixit BL, Raha T, Green MR, Tissenbaum HA. Identification of direct DAF-16 targets controlling longevity, metabolism and diapause by chromatin immunoprecipitation. Nat Genet 2006;38:251–7.
53. Lee SS, Kennedy S, Tolonen AC, Ruvkun G. DAF-16 target genes that control *C. elegans* life-span and metabolism. Science 2003;300:644–7.
54. Murphy CT, McCarroll SA, Bargmann CI, et al. Genes that act downstream of DAF-16 to influence the lifespan of *Caenorhabditis elegans*. Nature 2003;424:277–83.
55. Lee SS, Lee RY, Fraser AG, Kamath RS, Ahringer J, Ruvkun G. A systematic RNAi screen identifies a critical role for mitochondria in *C. elegans* longevity. Nat Genet 2003;33:40–8.
56. Nakae J, Barr V, Accili D. Differential regulation of gene expression by insulin and IGF-1 receptors correlates with phosphorylation of a single amino acid residue in the forkhead transcription factor FKHR. EMBO J 2000;19:989–96.
57. Zhang X, Gan L, Pan H, et al. Phosphorylation of serine 256 suppresses transactivation by FKHR (FOXO1) by multiple mechanisms. Direct and indirect effects on nuclear/cytoplasmic shuttling and DNA binding. J Biol Chem 2002;277:45276–84.
58. Durham SK, Suwanichkul A, Scheimann AO, et al. FKHR binds the insulin response element in the insulin-like growth factor binding protein-1 promoter. Endocrinology 1999;140:3140–6.
59. Tang ED, Nunez G, Barr FG, Guan KL. Negative regulation of the forkhead transcription factor FKHR by Akt. J Biol Chem 1999;274:16741–6.
60. Yu H, Larsen PL. DAF-16-dependent and independent expression targets of DAF-2 insulin receptor-like pathway in *Caenorhabditis elegans* include FKBPs. J Mol Biol 2001;314:1017–28.
61. McElwee J, Bubb K, Thomas JH. Transcriptional outputs of the *Caenorhabditis elegans* forkhead protein DAF-16. Aging Cell 2003;2:111–21.
62. McCarroll SA, Murphy CT, Zou S, et al. Comparing genomic expression patterns across species identifies shared transcriptional profile in aging. Nat Genet 2004;36:197–204.
63. Nasrin N, Ogg S, Cahill CM, et al. DAF-16 recruits the CREB-binding protein coactivator complex to the insulin-like growth factor binding protein 1 promoter in HepG2 cells. Proc Natl Acad Sci U S A 2000;97:10412–7.
64. Hall RK, Yamasaki T, Kucera T, Waltner-Law M, O'Brien R, Granner DK. Regulation of phosphoenolpyruvate carboxykinase and insulin-like growth factor-binding protein-1 gene expression by insulin. The role of winged helix/forkhead proteins. J Biol Chem 2000;275:30169–75.
65. Ambros V, Bartel B, Bartel DP, et al. A uniform system for microRNA annotation. RNA 2003;9(3):277–9.
66. Schmoll D, Walker KS, Alessi DR, et al. Regulation of glucose-6-phosphatase gene expression by protein kinase Balpha and the forkhead transcription factor FKHR. Evidence for insulin response unit-dependent and -independent effects of insulin on promoter activity. J Biol Chem 2000;275:36324–33.
67. Oh SW, Mukhopadhyay A, Svrzikapa N, Jiang F, Davis RJ, Tissenbaum HA. JNK regulates lifespan in *Caenorhabditis elegans* by modulating nuclear translocation of forkhead transcription factor/DAF-16. Proc Natl Acad Sci U S A 2005;102:4494–9.
68. Boehm M, Slack F. A developmental timing microRNA and its target regulate life span in *C. elegans*. Science 2005;310:1954–7.
69. Hallam SJ, Jin Y. lin-14 regulates the timing of synaptic remodelling in *Caenorhabditis elegans*. Nature 1998;395:78–82.
70. Ruvkun G, Giusto J. The *Caenorhabditis elegans* heterochronic gene lin-14 encodes a nuclear protein that forms a temporal developmental switch. Nature 1989;338:313–9.
71. Hong Y, Lee RC, Ambros V. Structure and function analysis of LIN-14, a temporal regulator of postembryonic developmental events in *Caenorhabditis elegans*. Mol Cell Biol 2000;20:2285–95.
72. Lee RC, Feinbaum RL, Ambros V. The *C. elegans* heterochronic gene lin-4 encodes small RNAs with antisense complementarity to lin-14. Cell 1993;75:843–54.

73. Wightman B, Ha I, Ruvkun G. Posttranscriptional regulation of the heterochronic gene lin-14 by lin-4 mediates temporal pattern formation in *C. elegans*. Cell 1993;75:855–62.
74. Bluher M, Michael MD, Peroni OD, et al. Adipose tissue selective insulin receptor knockout protects against obesity and obesity-related glucose intolerance. Dev Cell 2002;3:25–38.
75. Ren P, Lim CS, Johnsen R, Albert PS, Pilgrim D, Riddle DL. Control of *C. elegans* larval development by neuronal expression of a TGF-beta homolog. Science 1996;274:1389–91.
76. Georgi LL, Albert PS, Riddle DL. daf-1, a *C. elegans* gene controlling dauer larva development, encodes a novel receptor protein kinase. Cell 1990;61:635–45.
77. Estevez M, Attisano L, Wrana JL, Albert PS, Massague J, Riddle DL. The daf-4 gene encodes a bone morphogenetic protein receptor controlling *C. elegans* dauer larva development. Nature 1993;365:644–9.
78. Inoue T, Thomas J. Suppressors of transforming growth factor-beta pathway mutants in the *Caenorhabditis elegans* dauer formation pathway. Genetics 2000;156:1035–46.
79. Patterson GI, Koweek A, Wong A, Liu Y, Ruvkun G. The DAF-3 Smad protein antagonizes TGF-beta-related receptor signaling in the *Caenorhabditis elegans* dauer pathway. Genes Dev 1997;11:2679–90.
80. Shaw WM, Luo S, Landis J, Ashraf J, Murphy CT. The *C. elegans* TGF-beta Dauer pathway regulates longevity via insulin signaling. Curr Biol 2007;17:1635–45.
81. Wolkow CA, Kimura KD, Lee MS, Ruvkun G. Regulation of *C. elegans* life-span by insulinlike signaling in the nervous system. Science 2000;290:147–50.
82. Libina N, Berman J, Kenyon C. Tissue-specific activities of *C. elegans* DAF-16 in the regulation of lifespan. Cell 2003;115:489–502.
83. Murphy CT, Lee SJ, Kenyon C. Tissue entrainment by feedback regulation of insulin gene expression in the endoderm of *Caenorhabditis elegans*. Proc Natl Acad Sci U S A 2007;104:19046–50.
84. Pierce SB, Costa M, Wisotzkey R, et al. Regulation of DAF-2 receptor signaling by human insulin and ins-1, a member of the unusually large and diverse *C. elegans* insulin gene family. Genes Dev 2001;15:672–86.
85. Li W, Kennedy SG, Ruvkun G. daf-28 encodes a *C. elegans* insulin superfamily member that is regulated by environmental cues and acts in the DAF-2 signaling pathway. Genes Dev 2003;17:844–58.
86. Finch CE, Ruvkun G. The genetics of aging. Annu Rev Genomics Hum Genet 2001;2:435–62.
87. Libert S, Pletcher SD. Modulation of longevity by environmental sensing. Cell 2007;131:1231–4.
88. Alcedo J, Kenyon C. Regulation of *C. elegans* longevity by specific gustatory and olfactory neurons. Neuron 2004;41:45–55.
89. Lindemann B. Receptors and transduction in taste. Nature 2001;413:219–25.
90. Morley JF, Brignull HR, Weyers JJ, Morimoto RI. The threshold for polyglutamine-expansion protein aggregation and cellular toxicity is dynamic and influenced by aging in *Caenorhabditis elegans*. Proc Natl Acad Sci U S A 2002;99:10417–22.
91. Pinkston-Gosse J, Kenyon C. DAF-16/FOXO targets genes that regulate tumor growth in *Caenorhabditis elegans*. Nat Genet 2007;39:1403–9.
92. Seoane J, Le HV, Shen L, Anderson SA, Massague J. Integration of Smad and forkhead pathways in the control of neuroepithelial and glioblastoma cell proliferation. Cell 2004;117:211–23.
93. Brunet A, Bonni A, Zigmond MJ, et al. Akt promotes cell survival by phosphorylating and inhibiting a Forkhead transcription factor. Cell 1999;96:857–68.
94. Dijkers PF, Medema RH, Lammers JW, Koenderman L, Coffer PJ. Expression of the pro-apoptotic Bcl-2 family member Bim is regulated by the forkhead transcription factor FKHR-L1. Curr Biol 2000;10:1201–4.
95. Pinkston JM, Garigan D, Hansen M, Kenyon C. Mutations that increase the life span of *C. elegans* inhibit tumor growth. Science 2006;313:971–5.
96. Larsen P, Albert P, Riddle D. Genes that regulate both development and longevity in *Caenorhabditis elegans*. Genetics 1995;139:1567–83.
97. Gems D, Partridge L. Insulin/IGF signalling and ageing: seeing the bigger picture. Curr Opin Genet Dev 2001;11:287–92.

98. Snieder H, MacGregor AJ, Spector TD. Genes control the cessation of a woman's reproductive life: a twin study of hysterectomy and age at menopause. J Clin Endocrinol Metab 1998;83:1875–80.
99. Hsin H, Kenyon C. Signals from the reproductive system regulate the lifespan of *C. elegans*. Nature 1999;399:362–6.
100. Berman J, Kenyon C. Germ-cell loss extends *C. elegans* life span through regulation of DAF-16 by kri-1 and lipophilic-hormone signaling. Cell 2006;124:1055–68.
101. Cargill SL, Carey JR, Muller HG, Anderson G. Age of ovary determines remaining life expectancy in old ovariectomized mice. Aging Cell 2003;2:185–90.
102. Houthoofd K, Braeckman BP, Lenaerts I, et al. No reduction of metabolic rate in food restricted *Caenorhabditis elegans*. Exp Gerontol 2002;37:1359–69.
103. Lakowski B, Hekimi S. The genetics of caloric restriction in *Caenorhabditis elegans*. Proc Natl Acad Sci U S A 1998;95:13091–6.
104. Bartke A, Brown-Borg H. Life extension in the dwarf mouse. Curr Top Dev Biol 2004; 63:189–225.
105. Kaeberlein TL, Smith ED, Tsuchiya M, et al. Lifespan extension in *Caenorhabditis elegans* by complete removal of food. Aging Cell 2006;5:487–94.
106. Sohal RS, Weindruch R. Oxidative stress, caloric restriction, and aging. Science 1996; 273:59–63.
107. Houthoofd K, Braeckman BP, Johnson TE, Vanfleteren JR. Life extension via dietary restriction is independent of the Ins/IGF-1 signalling pathway in *Caenorhabditis elegans*. Exp Gerontol 2003;38:947–54.
108. Westphal CH, Dipp MA, Guarente L. A therapeutic role for sirtuins in diseases of aging? Trends Biochem Sci 2007;32(12):555–60.
109. Howitz KT, Bitterman KJ, Cohen HY, et al. Small molecule activators of sirtuins extend *Saccharomyces cerevisiae* lifespan. Nature 2003;425:191–6.
110. Wood JG, Rogina B, Lavu S, et al. Sirtuin activators mimic caloric restriction and delay ageing in metazoans. Nature 2004;430:686–9.
111. Tissenbaum HA, Guarente L. Increased dosage of a sir-2 gene extends lifespan in *Caenorhabditis elegans*. Nature 2001;410:227–30.
112. Wang Y, Tissenbaum H. Overlapping and distinct functions for a *Caenorhabditis elegans* SIR2 and DAF-16/FOXO. Mech Ageing Dev 2006;127:48–56.
113. Brunet A, Sweeney LB, Sturgill JF, et al. Stress-dependent regulation of FOXO transcription factors by the SIRT1 deacetylase. Science 2004;303:2011–5.
114. Daitoku H, Hatta M, Matsuzaki H, et al. Silent information regulator 2 potentiates Foxo1-mediated transcription through its deacetylase activity. Proc Natl Acad Sci U S A 2004;101:10042–7.
115. Kaeberlein M, Powers RW III, Steffen KK, et al. Regulation of yeast replicative life span by TOR and Sch9 in response to nutrients. Science 2005;310:1193–6.
116. Powers RW III, Kaeberlein M, Caldwell SD, Kennedy BK, Fields S. Extension of chronological life span in yeast by decreased TOR pathway signaling. Genes Dev 2006;20:174–84.
117. Jia K, Chen D, Riddle DL. The TOR pathway interacts with the insulin signaling pathway to regulate *C. elegans* larval development, metabolism and life span. Development 2004; 131:3897–906.
118. Vellai T, Takacs-Vellai K, Zhang Y, Kovacs AL, Orosz L, Muller F. Genetics: influence of TOR kinase on lifespan in C. elegans. Nature 2003;426:620.
119. Panowski S, Wolff S, Aguilaniu H, Durieux J, Dillin A. PHA-4/Foxa mediates diet-restriction-induced longevity of *C. elegans*. Nature 2007;447:550–5.
120. Bishop N, Guarente L. Two neurons mediate diet-restriction-induced longevity in *C. elegans*. Nature 2007;447:545–9.
121. Lakowski B, Hekimi S. Determination of life-span in *Caenorhabditis elegans* by four clock genes. Science 1996;272:1010–3.
122. Ewbank JJ, Barnes TM, Lakowski B, Lussier M, Bussey H, Hekimi S. Structural and functional conservation of the *Caenorhabditis elegans* timing gene clk-1. Science 1997; 275:980–3.

123. Jonassen T, Larsen PL, Clarke CF. A dietary source of coenzyme Q is essential for growth of long-lived *Caenorhabditis elegans* clk-1 mutants. Proc Natl Acad Sci U S A 2001; 98:421–6.
124. Miyadera H, Amino H, Hiraishi A, et al. Altered quinone biosynthesis in the long-lived clk-1 mutants of *Caenorhabditis elegans*. J Biol Chem 2001;276:7713–6.
125. Larsen PL, Clarke CF. Extension of life-span in *Caenorhabditis elegans* by a diet lacking coenzyme Q. Science 2002;295:120–3.
126. Liu X, Jiang N, Hughes B, Bigras E, Shoubridge E, Hekimi S. Evolutionary conservation of the clk-1-dependent mechanism of longevity: loss of mclk1 increases cellular fitness and lifespan in mice. Genes Dev 2005;19:2424–34.
127. Feng J, Bussiere F, Hekimi S. Mitochondrial electron transport is a key determinant of life span in *Caenorhabditis elegans*. Dev Cell 2001;1:633–44.
128. Dillin A, Hsu A, Arantes-Oliveira N, et al. Rates of behavior and aging specified by mitochondrial function during development. Science 2002;298:2398–401.
129. Ishii N, Fujii M, Hartman PS, et al. A mutation in succinate dehydrogenase cytochrome b causes oxidative stress and ageing in nematodes. Nature 1998;394:694–7.
130. Fire A, Xu S, Montgomery MK, Kostas SA, Driver SE, Mello CC. Potent and specific genetic interference by double-stranded RNA in *Caenorhabditis elegans*. Nature 1998;391:806–11.
131. Tabara H, Grishok A, Mello CC. RNAi in *C. elegans*: soaking in the genome sequence. Science 1998;282:430–1.
132. Timmons L, Court DL, Fire A. Ingestion of bacterially expressed dsRNAs can produce specific and potent genetic interference in *Caenorhabditis elegans*. Gene 2001;263:103–12.
133. Kamath RS, Fraser AG, Dong Y, et al. Systematic functional analysis of the *Caenorhabditis elegans* genome using RNAi. Nature 2003;421:231–7.
134. Rual JF, Ceron J, Koreth J, et al. Toward improving *Caenorhabditis elegans* phenome mapping with an ORFeome-based RNAi library. Genome Res 2004;14:2162–8.
135. van Ham TJ, Thijssen KL, Breitling R, Hofstra RM, Plasterk RH, Nollen EA. *C. elegans* model identifies genetic modifiers of alpha-synuclein inclusion formation during aging. PLoS Genet 2008;4:e1000027.
136. Brignull H, Morley J, Garcia S, Morimoto R. Modeling polyglutamine pathogenesis in *C. elegans*. Methods Enzymol 2006;412:256–82.
137. Hamilton B, Dong Y, Shindo M, et al. A systematic RNAi screen for longevity genes in *C. elegans*. Genes Dev 2005;19:1544–55.
138. Curran S, Ruvkun G. Lifespan regulation by evolutionarily conserved genes essential for viability. PLoS Genet 2007;3:e56.
139. Dillin A, Crawford D, Kenyon C. Timing requirements for insulin/IGF-1 signaling in *C. elegans*. Science 2002;298:830–4.
140. Hansen M, Hsu AL, Dillin A, Kenyon C. New genes tied to endocrine, metabolic, and dietary regulation of lifespan from a *Caenorhabditis elegans* genomic RNAi screen. PLoS Genet 2005;1:e17.
141. Lee SS. Whole genome RNAi screens for increased longevity: important new insights but not the whole story. Exp Gerontol 2006;41:968–73.
142. Williams PD, Day T. Antagonistic pleiotropy, mortality source interactions, and the evolutionary theory of senescence. Evolution 2003;57:1478–88.
143. Chen D, Pan KZ, Palter JE, Kapahi P. Longevity determined by developmental arrest genes in *Caenorhabditis elegans*. Aging Cell 2007;6:525–33.
144. Hansen M, Taubert S, Crawford D, Libina N, Lee S, Kenyon C. Lifespan extension by conditions that inhibit translation in *Caenorhabditis elegans*. Aging Cell 2007;6:95–110.
145. Hipkiss A. On why decreasing protein synthesis can increase lifespan. Mech Ageing Dev 2007;128:412–4.
146. Samuelson AV, Carr CE, Ruvkun G. Gene activities that mediate increased life span of *C. elegans* insulin-like signaling mutants. Genes Dev 2007;21:2976–94.
147. Melendez A, Talloczy Z, Seaman M, Eskelinen EL, Hall DH, Levine B. Autophagy genes are essential for dauer development and life-span extension in *C. elegans*. Science 2003;301:1387–91.

148. Wolff S, Ma H, Burch D, Maciel G, Hunter T, Dillin A. SMK-1, an essential regulator of DAF-16-mediated longevity. Cell 2006;124:1039–53.
149. Melov S, Ravenscroft J, Malik S, et al. Extension of life-span with superoxide dismutase/catalase mimetics. Science 2000;289:1567–9.
150. Evason K, Collins JJ, Huang C, Hughes S, Kornfeld K. Valproic acid extends *Caenorhabditis elegans* lifespan. Aging Cell 2008;7:305–17.
151. Zou S, Sinclair J, Wilson MA, et al. Comparative approaches to facilitate the discovery of prolongevity interventions: effects of tocopherols on lifespan of three invertebrate species. Mech Ageing Dev 2007;128:222–6.
152. Evason K, Huang C, Yamben I, Covey DF, Kornfeld K. Anticonvulsant medications extend worm life-span. Science 2005;307:258–62.
153. Wilson MA, Shukitt-Hale B, Kalt W, Ingram DK, Joseph JA, Wolkow CA. Blueberry polyphenols increase lifespan and thermotolerance in *Caenorhabditis elegans*. Aging Cell 2006;5:59–68.
154. Petrascheck M, Ye X, Buck LB. An antidepressant that extends lifespan in adult Caenorhabditis elegans. Nature 2007;450:553–6.
155. Baur JA, Pearson KJ, Price NL, et al. Resveratrol improves health and survival of mice on a high-calorie diet. Nature 2006;444:337–42.

# Part III
# *Drosophila melanogaster*

# Chapter 4
# The Genetic Architecture of Longevity

**Robert Arking**

**Abstract** Longevity is a more complex process than is often thought. The adult life span can be naturally partitioned into two phases: the health span and the senescence span. The transition between them is characterized by the downward inflection of the survival curve. The evidence shows that there are three ways to increase longevity, only one of which involves an increase in the values of both mean and maximum life spans. In that case, the extra longevity is expressed as an extension of the health span, whereas the senescent span is little affected if at all. The delayed onset of senescence phenotype is the most desirable way of extending the life span. This multiphasic view of the life span is supported by a variety of literature data and springs from an evolutionary view of the aging process. Gene activity during the life span can best be viewed in terms of gene networks, their progressive increase in fidelity during development, their maintenance during much of the health span, their progressive loss of stringent feedback control as the force of natural selection wanes, and the stochastic destabilization of key cellular functions during the senescent phase. This systems biology overview should be of conceptual value in understanding the biology of specific long-lived mutants and selected strains.

**Keywords** Life span • health span • senescent span • gene network • genetic architecture of longevity • *Drosophila*

**Abbreviations** DOS: Delayed onset of senescence; MEMN: Macrophage-enriched metabolic network; PD: Population doubling; QTL: Quantitative trait loci; SNP: Single nucleotide polymorphism

---

R. Arking
Department of Biological Sciences, BSB 3103, Wayne State University, Detroit, MI, 48085, USA
e-mail: aa2210@wayne.edu

C. Sell et al. (eds.), *Life-Span Extension,* Aging Medicine,
DOI 10.1007/978-1-60327-507-1_4,

## 4.1 The Three Types of Longevity Responses

Longevity is a more complex process than one that merely allows the addition or subtraction of time to the end of some relatively stable life span. None of society's earlier efforts to increase life span had anything to do with altering the aging process. This observation may seem contradictory in view of the fact that one of the great achievements of the twentieth century was the ~60% increase in mean life span that took place in developed countries. But that increase was the result of public and individual health interventions that had everything to do with improving the human environment, thereby decreasing the premature mortality inherent in a harsh environment. It resulted in a significant increase of the mean life span but not of the maximum life span; and it achieved these successes because it removed the extrinsic causes of death. It did not, however, affect the intrinsic causes (i.e., slow the aging process) and thus increase the maximum life span. Our ability to manipulate the processes of aging in the laboratory and significantly increase the maximum life span of our model systems has been laboriously developed only over the past 25 years or so, and their elucidation was made possible only when investigators used evolutionary principles to uncover them.

The lives of animals can be lengthened in three ways: increasing both their mean and maximum life span; increasing their mean but not their maximum life span; or increasing their maximum but not their mean life span (Fig. 4.1a–c) ***(1)***. Although each of the three treatments resulted in a significant alteration of the survival curves, only the first treatment resulted in a significant slowing of the age-specific mortality rate (Fig. 4.2a–c). The latter two approaches transiently decreased the mortality rate only at the beginning or end of life, and neither case represents an optimal increase of healthy life span. Only the first approach caused the organism to enhance its existing repair and maintenance capabilities so as to actually slow the aging rate and thereby delay the onset of senescence.

The three longevity types are probably general, in the sense that they exhaust the logical permutations of variations in the mortality curves. The fact that one might have to use different variants of the basic Gompertz curve to best describe the data or that different genomes might well use the same stimulus (or variants of the same stimulus) to induce different responses does not detract from the general applicability of these three major longevity types. There is no reason to believe that this one strain is special and every reason to believe that many if not all wild-type strains in this and other species are capable of mounting the same set of responses. The presence of three alternative longevity phenotypes in the same organism means that the genetic mechanisms regulating longevity are more complex than is often assumed ***(2)***.

The delayed onset of senescence (DOS) phenotype shown in Figs. 4.1a and 4.2a would clearly be the desired outcome for an eventual longevity intervention in humans. This desirability arises from the fact that the delay of the inflection point results in an extended health span while having minimal effect on the length of the senescent span (Fig. 4.2). The extra longevity is added to the health span and not to the senescent span; this observation suggests that the adult life span is based on a multiphasic genetic architecture (Table 4.1). The existence of a complex architecture

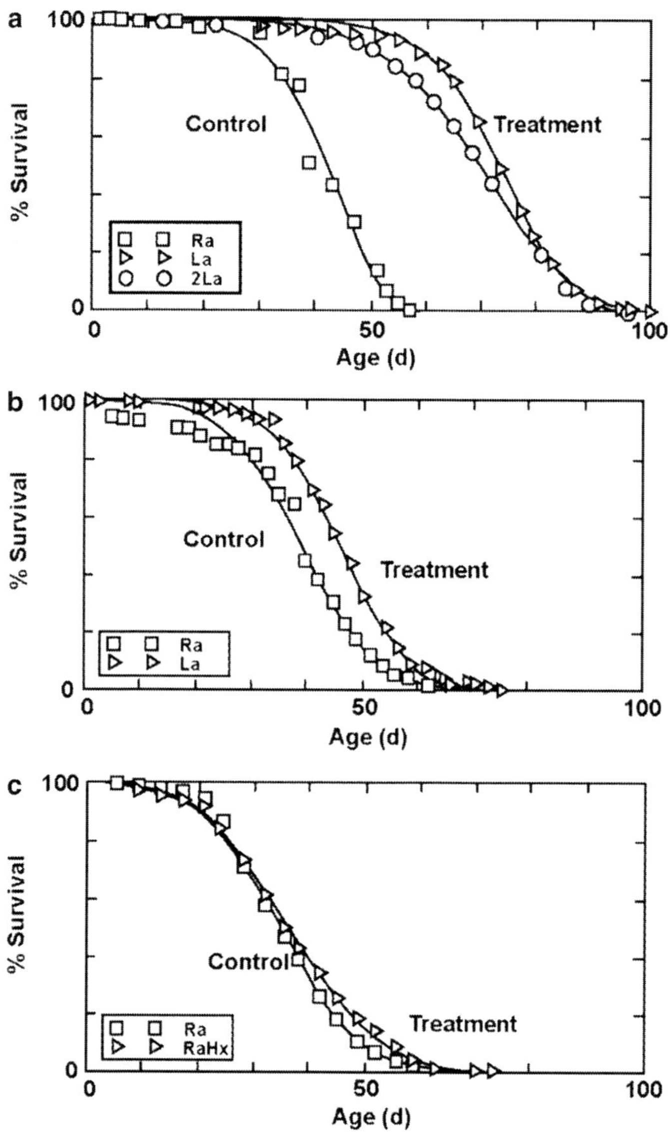


**Fig. 4.1** The three ways of altering mortality kinetics and thus longevity in *Drosophila*. It is assumed that these alterations are generally applicable to other species as well. Three different types of survival curves: (**a**) an increase in both mean and maximum life span; (**b**) an increase in mean but not in maximum life span; (**c**) an increase in maximum but not in mean life span. La and 2La are two long-lived *Drosophila* strains; Ra is a normal-lived strain; and RaHx is a heat-treated strain. From Arking et al. *(1)*. Copyright © The Gerontological Society of America. Reproduced by permission publisher

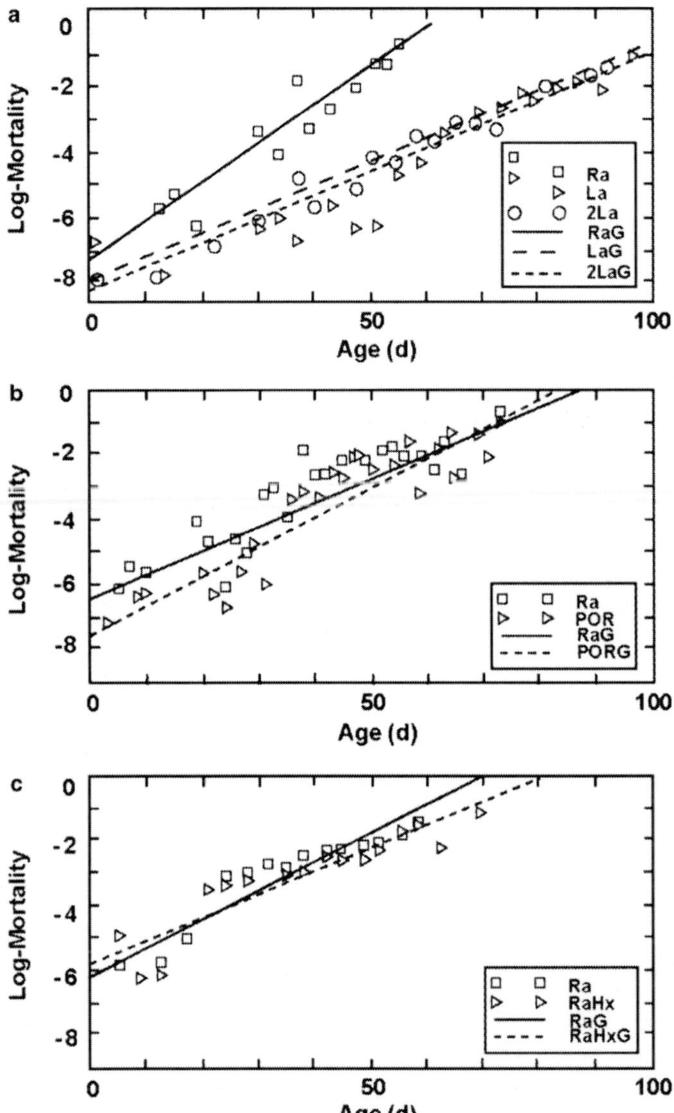


**Fig. 4.2** Three different types of age-specific mortality curves corresponding to the three survival curves of Fig. 4.1. The mortality kinetics were altered in one of the three different ways to yield the corresponding survival curves: (**a**) for the survival curves of Fig. 4.1a, the age-specific mortality rate is lower throughout the entire life span; (**b**) for the survival curves of Fig. 4.1b, the age-specific mortality rate is lower in early life but increases in late life; and (**c**) for the survival curves of Fig. 4.1c, the age-specific mortality curve is higher in early life but lower in later life. La and 2La are two long-lived *Drosophila* strains; POR is a paraquat-resistant strain; and RaHx is a heat-treated strain. "G" denotes Gompertz approximations of the data points. From Arking et al. *(1)*. Copyright © The Gerontological Society of America. Reproduced by permission of the publisher

**Table 4.1** Overview of the changes in gene expression and architecture during the developmental, health, and senescent phases of the life span as well as during the transition phase between the latter two spans

| Developmental span | Health span | Transition phase | Senescent span |
|---|---|---|---|
| Gene network innately differentiates but can be perturbed by maternal or developmental effects | Gene-dependent longevity assurance mechanisms operative | Event- and history-dependent loss of optimal function | Stochastic effects on unique genome lead to loss of function |
| Gene/protein interaction networks differentiate via developmental program | Gene/protein interaction networks are at optimal levels but are sensitive to epigenetic (e.g., nutrition) perturbation | Altered balance of cell's defenses due to accumulated damage and/or loss of intercellular or intracellular signals | Degradation of gene/protein interaction networks brought on by spoke gene perturbation of gene network dynamic equilibrium |
| Cell replication and body growth dominant activities | Longevity determinant mechanisms operative; cells are in growth/reproduction mode but still have high levels of repair and maintenance | Timing and nature of transition may be influenced by cell network states induced during development | Cell's regulatory ability decreases due to suboptimal expression within or between cells |
| Cells in some systems (neural, metabolic) may be perturbed into other long-term equilibrium states by pre- and/or postnatal events | Homeostatic ability sensitive and reliable | Abnormal proteins aggregate, exceed chaperone capacity; damage accumulates and initiates a positive feedback of damage induction; yields lowered cell function | Tissue and/or systemic functions deteriorate due to increase in senescent cells within tissues and/or to decreased replicative ability of tissue-specific stem cells |
| | | Damaged cells survive, apoptosis decreases, tumors increase | Positive feedback damage cascades lessen cell's homeostatic ability; tissue function suffers |
| Minimum age-specific mortality rate reached just prior to sexual maturation | Cells have sufficient reserve capacity to deal with various stressors | Age-specific mortality rate may show sharp increase | Critical thresholds are passed; cell function ceases |

implies the possibility of multiple points at which one might intervene in the life span and further raises the possibility that the several phases may be lightly connected and thus susceptible to different stimuli. Our analysis of the data from our laboratory as well as of that from the literature leads us to support these predictions. This unexpected expression of an induced healthy longevity has public policy implications very different from those mistakenly foreseen by almost all political leaders, and I have dealt with that topic elsewhere ***(3)***. A more detailed analysis of the DOS phenotype is provided in Fig. 4.2.

## 4.2 The Three Phases of the Life Span

### *4.2.1 The Developmental Span*

The developmental phase covers the period of time from conception to the age when the young becomes calorically self-sufficient and therefore able to effectively reproduce. Analysis of the human anthropologic data of various hunter–gatherer tribes leads to the conclusion that our development span covers the period from conception to ~18 to 20 years and is energetically very expensive (~$12.6 \times 10^9$ kcal) ***(4)***. Higher levels of fecundity in humans are associated with decreased survival of parents ***(5)*** and/or an alteration in the iconic life history of children developing in energetically challenging environments ***(6, 7)***. Analysis of human age-specific mortality rates shows that aging, understood as an increased probability of dying with increased age, does not begin until the onset of puberty at ~10 years of age [see Fig. 2.16 in ***(3)***] ***(8)***. Prenatal development is clearly understood to be a program in the sense that development consists of a series of gene expression modules in which the output of one module is the input for the next ***(9, 10)***. Developmental gene expression patterns for any species are highly complex yet very predictable in that they depend almost entirely on the nature of the *cis*-acting regulatory elements of the genes involved ***(11)***. They may be viewed as leading to a stage of highest optimal functionality at or about puberty, as judged by the minimum values of the age-specific mortality rate. Although development is mostly internally driven, chance may still play an important role in individuals ***(12)***. These developmental expression patterns are susceptible to certain environmental influences affecting their basic regulatory mechanisms and thus altering their future life span ***(13–15)***. For this reason, the developmental phase of the life span cannot be excluded when considering the overall genetic architecture of longevity.

### *4.2.2 The Health Span*

The end of growth and development ushers in the health span, which is defined by a low age-specific mortality rate and a high survival rate. The health span ends when the age-specific mortality rate begins to increase significantly or when the survival rate drops below 90%. The negative inflection in the survival curve at this point indicates the transition between the health span and the senescent span, the two obviously different phases of the adult life span. The question arises as to whether these two phases are actually separable or whether they are perhaps simply different portions of the same continuum. Biomarker studies ***(16)*** showed that the processes taking place during the senescent phases of both the normal- and long-lived strains occurred at the same relative stages, indicating that senescence in both strains involved the same processes and took a similar length of time in the life cycle of both. On the other hand, the same biomarker analysis showed that the health spans of the two strains differed both functionally and temporally. The long-lived strain expressed an early specific upregulation of multiple antioxidant scavenger enzymes that was absent in the normal-lived strain ***(17, 18)*** and that was shown to have a causal relationship with DOS ***(19)***. The two phases are separable, having different gene expression patterns and physiological functions. Longevity is not just one long process of erosion but rather a complex process in which different stimuli can give rise to alternate patterns of gene expression that give rise via differential mortality to the three longevity phenotypes of Fig. 4.1. Our long-lived La strain of *Drosophila* lives longer because its health span has been genetically altered, not because its senescent span is different in any way.

Much discussion is available about aging mechanisms, but this term lumps together processes involved in our health span with those mostly involved in our senescent span. We have shown that the health span can be regulated independently of the senescent span, which means that the mechanisms involved are not necessarily continuous from one phase to the other, so they should be separated for clarity of thought. Separating them makes it clear that the two aspects of the life span have qualitatively different types of mechanisms operative.

The available data strongly suggest that the mechanisms operative during the health span are primarily genetic in origin and are under the influence of natural selection. This concept should not be considered simply a modern form of genetic determinism; the fact that longevity responds to the environment makes it clear that it is the outcome of a complex gene–environment interaction. Identifying the standard environmental conditions necessary for that gene expression, as well as the environmental variables that alter the standard expression ***(20)***, allows the slow reintegration of genotype and environment as covariables in the expression of a complex phenotype.

Laboratory experiments have allowed the robust identification of four different – but intertwined – groups of genetic and physiological pathways that seem to regulate longevity in all of the major animal model systems. These have been explained in detail elsewhere (Chapter 7 of ref 3) and show that aging is a cell-level phenomenon. The pathways include several different high-level intercellular integrative processes (sensory and neuroendocrine) that regulate intracellular signal transduction pathways (e.g., insulin-like signaling pathway, target of rapamycin, c-Jun N-terminal kinase) that affect upstream regulatory genes and downstream target genes. These effects are modulated by intraorganismal tissue competition (gonads vs. somatic cells); the effectiveness of essential supporting processes (DNA repair); and organelle interactions (retrograde regulation or nuclear–mitochondrial interactions), which together give rise to the observed longevity phenotype.

If we describe these mechanisms in terms of the gene expression networks discussed in Sect. 4.2.3, we can view these several longevity determinant mechanisms as epigenetically induced alterations in the activity of a network gene that perturbs its own subnetwork to shift from a stable dynamic equilibrium favoring growth and reproduction to another type of stable dynamic equilibrium favoring somatic repair and maintenance. The DOS phenotype depends on the latter type of genomic state. We have shown that the longevity of the Ra animals can be mathematically modeled as an exercise in optimal resource allocation between reproduction effort and somatic maintenance efforts ***(21)***.

The long-lived animals are characterized by high levels of damage prevention and prophylactic repair. These positive effects are counterbalanced by the gradual buildup of unrepaired cell and/or tissue damage. The damage itself may only be a proximal cause of senescence. The actual underlying cause may be the decline in the force of natural selection as the reproductive period ends ***(22, 23)***. Nonetheless, senescence manifests itself in the form of unrepaired damage that exceeds various tissue-specific critical thresholds and so senescence ensues.

### *4.2.3 The Senescent Span*

Senescence involves the loss of function. It is this portion of the life span that is commonly referred to by the word aging. Humans and the common laboratory model organisms used to study senescence are all species that undergo a gradual senescence. The canonical patterns of senescence in these species were elucidated by Finch [Table 1.1 in ***(24)***] as encompassing most or all of the following: mortality acceleration, reproductive decline, slowed movements, cardiovascular dysfunctions, abnormal growths, oxidative damage, and neuron loss.

What exactly happens to individual animals at the inflection point of the survival curves in Fig. 4.2 that increases their age-specific mortality rate and decreases their functional ability in such canonical patterns? From an evolutionary viewpoint, the optimal life history is weighted toward early performance at the expense of late performance, which it achieves through some optimal resource allocation between reproduction and somatic maintenance ***(21)***. A conceptual explanation presented by Arking [Table 4.1 in ***(3)***] suggested that the gene networks that maintain our bodily functions at an optimal (or near optimal) level during our health span gradually lose their internal connectivity as a result of genetic and environmental effects. These destabilizing effects may be the visible aspects of the decline in the force of natural selection as the reproductive period ends ***(22, 23)***. Such effects may take the form of decreased fidelity in feedback control with a consequently increased variance in multiple processes, leading to an increased probability of external perturbation of the network. These perturbations in network efficiencies may lead to the accumulation of unrepaired damage, a loss of diverse functions, and thus to the transition into the senescent phase. Should the damages involve multiple systems, then there need not be any one universal cause of senescence.

Senescence is not a programmed response in the same sense as is embryonic development; nor is it a totally random process, for even though it is highly individualistic, common elements are present in many individuals. Senescence has many characteristics of a stochastic progressive loss of function but one that is somehow restrained in its apparent paths and outcomes. How can one explain both the apparent similarity and individuality of senescence among all humans without a genetic program? Of course, similar genomes in similar environments may well have similar constraints on their possible modes of failure, and so they may appear as canonical patterns of senescence. We can, however, go beyond this general statement. Many studies show that genomes can be best visualized as forming gene–gene interaction networks. Genes do not act by themselves but rather as one component of an integrated gene circuit or gene interaction network ***(9, 10, 25)***. Such networks are nonhomogeneous, which means that most genes have few connections, whereas others are highly connected. In other words, our gene interaction networks are hub (high connectivity) and spoke (low connectivity) networks in which the loss of an individual spoke gene will have a minor effect but in which the loss of a hub gene will have a major effect. Mendelian genes are major, or hub, genes and modifier genes are minor, or spoke, genes. Data from both animal and human studies ***(26, 27)*** indicate that senescence begins not with the inactivation of the major or Mendelian genes but with the stochastic loss of connectivity of individual spoke or modifier genes. Stochastic events, such as tissue-specific somatic mutations, lead to a decreased age-related connectivity of modifier genes. Although individual modifier genes have a small effect by themselves, collectively they account for most of the normal variance in the phenotype. For example, the eight specific Mendelian mutations that lead to human hypertension are modified by 107 quantitative trait loci (QTL) scattered over every chromosome ***(28)***. Given that these QTLs are presumably arranged in a network configuration, then the stochastic deregulation of the 107 spoke loci may have additive or even synergistic effects on blood pressure, leading to age-related hypertension in the absence of any mutational effect on the eight Mendelian hub genes. When the accumulated unrepaired damage reaches a threshold at which it saturates the cell's stress-resistance ability (i.e., no more reserve capacity), then any further accumulation of such damage will push the cell off its equilibrium point and into a positive feedback cascade in which each increment of damage causes a further loss of function. The organism shifts from its health span into its senescent span.

What are the mechanisms that result in the stochastic deregulation of spoke genes? A spectrum of such potential mechanisms exists. Weiss ***(29)*** developed a case for the idea that somatic mutation might be the cause of sporadically occurring but complex human diseases with a weak genetic signature. The plausibility of this hypothesis depends on the presence of relevant biological and epidemiological parameters, such as the etiology of the disease being due to aberrant gene action and a mechanism for expansion of the number of at-risk cells. He used idiopathic epilepsy as an example of such a disease, whereby an early occurring somatic mutation affecting ion channels (for example) is exponentially expanded by the number of mitoses required to construct the large number ($\sim 5 \times 10^7$) of neurons in the human brain. Variations in the penetrance or expressivity of the disease may be attributed to the date of origin of the somatic mutation and the morphological details of its expansion during development but not to any characteristics of the germ-line DNA.

Note that in the somatic mutation model, the genes are presumed to act alone, as in the classic model of gene action. We now know, however, that the genes are organized in a network, as described above. So how does a mutant or disease susceptibility variant act when it is embedded in a network? In fact, it turns out to be very difficult to definitively associate a single gene with a disease susceptibility, much less than a whole network of them. Two simultaneous reports have described the use of gene network analysis as an alternative to the traditional forward genetic protocols. Chen et al. ***(30)*** assayed a population of segregating recombinant inbred mice and assayed the behavior in them of obesity gene networks that could be significantly perturbed by known obesity susceptibility loci on chromosome 1 and so express the obesity phenotype. Liver- and adipose tissue-specific coexpression networks were constructed from the segregating mouse data and were correlated with the observed metabolic phenotypes. The correlations were more significant with the adipose tissue. A macrophage-enriched metabolic network (MEMN) of 1,350 genes was identified that was enriched for 207 genes affecting 14 gene ontology classifications significantly correlated with obesity and obesity-related diseases, including the inflammatory and immune responses. Substituting mutants for three of the 207 wild-type genes led to perturbations of the entire network, leading to the expression of an obese phenotype in the affected mice. Chen et al. [***(30)***, p. 434] concluded that "…common forms of disease may be emergent properties of networks, when the networks associated with disease are highly interconnected, with many genes in the network potentially having a causal relationship with disease if perturbed strongly enough." In the companion paper, Emilsson et al. ***(31)*** identified the same MEMN in blood and adipose tissue of both mice and humans. They tested the role of genetic variations on network expression by identifying the single nucleotide polymorphisms (SNPs) in the vicinity of each gene in the human MNEN network and correlated their expression with the individual's body mass index and percent body fat. The analysis of 768 cis eSNPs in 8,685 individuals showed a significant correlation with the individual's body mass index, a fact suggesting that genetic variation could alter the network dynamics. This finding was substantiated in the mouse by assaying the effect of two separate adipose-specific knockout genes (*Alox5* and *Hsd11b1*) and noting that each one significantly perturbed the MEMN expression pattern.

Finch ***(24)*** argues that the general senescence processes may be viewed as constituting three interacting suites of mechanisms: (a) physiological set points for food intake, physical activity, and hormone levels; (b) oxidant damage and inflammation; and (c) damage to irreplaceable cells and molecules. The gene network data summarized here deal with the first two of these suites. The general architecture of the gene network probably predicts the various set points in a general fashion, whereas the individual's specific genetic and epigenetic variables probably fine tune them into an individual profile. But the network data per se do not explicitly deal with the effects of loss of irreplaceable cells and molecules.

Stem cell loss may well be the most important factor affecting loss of somatic cells, particularly in long-lived species. The importance of tissue-specific stem cells as a source of new cells is now appreciated *(32)*. The aging of stem cells is expressed as a gradual decline in their replicative ability. This loss of replacement cells results in a demographic shift of the age structure of the cells that comprise the affected tissue. This shift from a situation in which the cell replacement rate equals the cell death rate to one in which the replacement rate is much less than the death rate results in an increasing proportion of reproductively senescent cells in the tissue. It is well known that senescent cells exhibit significant alterations in their gene expression patterns and their synthetic and metabolic activities. Their gene expression networks have been irreversibly perturbed. At least two excellent examples of the dysfunction brought about in different tissues by this demographic shift are available. Funk et al. *(33)* constructed human skin equivalents by using fibroblasts and keratinocytes obtained from an in vitro population of a defined population-doubling (PD) age and then subjected the reconstructed skin to a mechanical stress test. Skin constructed with PD20 (young) cells passed the stress test whereas skin constructed with PD60 (old) or PD80 (very old) cells failed the test, splitting apart at the junction of the laminin 5 and collagen VII extracellular matrix layers. Synthetic skin made from PD120 cells transgenic for telomerase activity was as resilient as PD20 normal skin. Normal skin has desmosomes at this junction; the assumption was that the old cells did not have them due to altered synthetic activities whereas the transgenic cells did have them thanks to their high telomerase activity. In another example, Torella et al. *(34)* demonstrated that cardiac function in the mouse was a function of cardiac cell age structure in the tissue. They took advantage of the fact that, within the heart, high levels of insulin-like growth factor I stimulate the cardiac stem cells to replicate. They constructed a transgenic mouse mutant that did just this and compared it to the normal control with respect to mitochondrial damage levels as well as rates of cell senescence and organ function. In the normal heart, the number of dead and dying cells far exceeded the number of newly formed cells; in the transgenic animals, the two populations were in balance. As a result, the normal heart gained in weight even while its cell number decreased, an outcome of the fact that senescent cells are significantly larger than young cells. The normal heart also became stiffer as a result of altered extracellular matrix syntheses and so lost function. In contrast, the transgenic heart cells showed a significantly smaller size increase whereas its cell numbers and functional status stayed about the same. Thus, enhanced stem cell activity, whether stimulated by exercise *(35)* or by transgenic means in mouse hearts, is an effective method of maintaining function for a longer time and hence delaying the onset of senescence.

The data discussed above allow us to conclude that a genetic (or epigenetic) perturbation of a complex of closely linked QTLs will interact with environmental effects (e.g., nutrition, exercise) to yield a perturbation of the larger gene network in such a manner as to potentially lead to continued optimal performance or to expression of the age-related senescent diseases such as diabetes. The gene network is adversely affected by the replicative senescence of the cell. The shutdown of the cell's reproductive ability, presumably brought about by specific cell signaling proteins (e.g., p16, etc.) as an evolved defense against cancer, cascades into an apparently severe perturbation of the cell's gene network expression pattern such that senescent cells can no longer maintain an optimal synthesis of important cell products. The failure of individual cells alters the functional ability of their tissue via both direct (altered cell age structure) and indirect [altered intercellular signaling ***(36)***] effects.

## 4.3 The Genetic Architecture of Longevity

The developmental span begins with the establishment and differentiation of the cell's interaction network and ends with the cell's gene expression networks functioning at optimal or near optimal levels in each of the several hundred different cell types that comprise our body. This span begins as a deterministic genetic program yielding intrinsically determined and controlled products. The emerging complexity of the offspring allows for the introduction of nondeterministic variables such as variations in maternal nutrition or behavior ***(13, 24)*** that can epigenetically affect the developing expression networks into establishing unexpected stable dynamic equilibria. The optimal functioning characteristic of fully developed young organisms continues into the health span but is shadowed by the slow buildup of unrepaired cell and molecular damage that is the inevitable consequence of the declining force of natural selection. Maintaining the integrity of the gene expression networks is critical to delaying the onset of senescence. Because the normal evolutionary pressures are to increase the individual's Darwinian fitness by reproducing, there is no selective advantage outside the laboratory for organisms to spend much energy on maintenance relative to reproduction ***(37)***. The loosening of the force of natural selection and the consequent buildup of unrepaired damage eventually cause the organism to transition from the health span to the senescent span, where both intrinsic and extrinsic variables so perturb the cell's gene expression networks that they lose function rapidly. The tissues that these senescent cells comprise lose function. These losses begin at the gene expression level but eventually are expressed in functional terms, such as the loss of specific behaviors, e.g., in flies, loss of negative geotactic or positive phototropic behaviors ***(38)***. They can be quantitatively expressed in demographic terms for humans, such as in the loss of the abilities of daily living in humans ***(39)*** or in the loss of physical strength ***(40)***, both of which are known predictors of mortality. The organism's functional ability eventually drops below some critical threshold, and the organism dies as a result of the failure of the first critical system that fails.

Our selected La strain animals are very robust compared with some single gene longevity mutants or certain weak wild-type strains. Our data suggest that one source of this observed robustness is the animal's reliance on upregulating multiple physiological processes to achieve its extended longevity [***(1)***; unpublished data]. The La strain relies on at least four upregulated processes for its extended health span. Network theory suggests that modular networks are robust networks; perhaps the same principle applies as well to genomes.

An integrated view of the life span incorporating the data and concepts discussed herein is presented in Fig. 4.3, which may be viewed as an overview of the genetic architecture of longevity. It is the task of future researchers to flesh out this figure with a full systems biology description and analysis of the changes in the gene expression networks that are important to our understanding of health and senescence. Current studies of genetic variants contributing to human disease find a multiplicity of weak variants with no as-yet clear idea of their mode of action ***(41)***. An intriguing clue is presented by the findings of Ruan and Wu ***(42)*** showing that flies homozygous for the cSOD$^{n1}$ (CuZn superoxide dismutase) mutation displayed an increased life span plus improved stress resistance and motor ability when they were cohoused with young helper flies of a different genotype. These observations raised the possibility that social interactions might also be able to somehow perturb a gene interaction network into a state conducive to extended longevity. It is possible that the overview of the genomic architecture presented here might offer a conceptual framework for understanding how such weak variants and/or social interactions could affect the systems biology of such a long-lived organism.

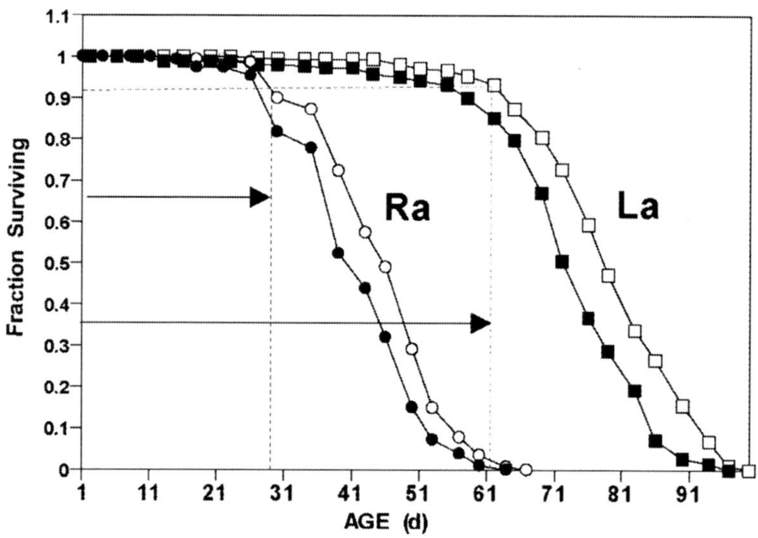


**Fig. 4.3** Survival curves of replicate populations of the normal-lived Ra flies (*circles*) and the long-lived La flies (*squares*). The *upper, shorter arrow* indicates the health span, defined as the time period in which a survival rate of ≥90% of the Ra flies is ~30 days; their senescent span, defined as the rest of the life span, is ~31 days. The *lower, longer arrow* indicates the health span of the La flies. The health span and senescent span values for the La flies are ~61 and ~35 days, respectively. Thus the extra life span induced by selection is added to the healthy portion of the life span rather than to the senescent phase (two replicates illustrate repeatability of the data)

## References


1. Arking R, Novoseltseva J, Hwangbo DS, et al. Different age-specific demographic profiles are generated in the same normal-lived *Drosophila* strain by different longevity stimuli. J Gerontol A Biol Sci Med Sci 2002;57:B390–8.
2. Barja G. The gene cluster hypothesis of aging and longevity. Biogerontology 2008;9:57–66.
3. Arking R. The biology of aging: observations and principles, 3rd ed. New York, NY: Oxford University Press, 2006.
4. Arking R. Human reproductive costs and the predicted response to dietary restriction. Rejuvenation Res 2007;10:11–9.
5. Penn DJ, Smith KR. Differential fitness costs of reproduction between the sexes. Proc Natl Acad Sci U S A 2007;104:553–8.
6. Larke A, Crews DE. Parental investment, late reproduction, and increased reserve capacity are associated with longevity in humans. J Physiol Anthropol 2006;25:119–31.
7. Walker R, Gurven M, Hill K, et al. Growth rate and life histories in twenty-two small-scale societies. Am J Hum Biol 2006;18:295–311.
8. Milne E. When does human ageing begin? Mech Ageing Dev 2006;127:290.
9. Davidson EH, Rast JP, Oliveri P. A provisional regulatory gene network for specification of endomesoderm in the sea urchin embryo. Dev Biol 2002;246:162–90.
10. Davidson EH, Erwin DH. Gene regulatory networks and the evolution of animal body plans. Science 2006;311:796–800.
11. Segal E, Raveh-Sadka T, Schroeder M, Unnerstall U, Gaul U. Predicting expression patterns from regulatory sequence in *Drosophila* segmentation. Nature 2008;451:535–40.
12. Finch CE, Kirkwood TBL. Chance, development, and aging. New York, NY: Oxford University Press, 2000.
13. Barker DJP. Intrauterine programming of adult disease. Mol Med Today 1995;1:418–23.
14. Baker KD, Thummel CS. Diabetic larvae and obese flies – emerging studies of metabolism in *Drosophila.* Cell Metab 2007;6:257–66.
15. Danese A, Pariante CM, Caspi A, Taylor A, Poultan R. Childhood maltreatment predicts adult inflammation in a life-course study. Proc Natl Acad Sci U S A 2007;104:1319–24.
16. Arking R, Wells RA. Genetic alteration of normal aging processes is responsible for extended longevity in *Drosophila*. Dev Genet 1990;11:141–8.
17. Dudas SP, Arking R. A coordinate up-regulation of antioxidant gene activities is required prior to the delayed onset of senescence characteristic of a long-lived strain of *Drosophila*. J Gerontol A Biol Sci Med Sci 1995;50A:B117–27.
18. Hari R, Burde V, Arking R. Immunological confirmation of elevated levels of CuZn superoxide dismutase protein in an artificially selected long-lived strain of *Drosophila melanogaster.* Exp Gerontol 1998;33:227–37.
19. Arking R, Burde V, Graves K, et al. Forward and reverse selection for longevity in *Drosophila* is characterized by alteration of antioxidant gene expression and oxidative damage patterns. Exp Gerontol 2000;35:167–85.
20. Libert S, Pletcher SD. Modulation of longevity by environmental sensing. Cell 2007;131:1231–4.
21. Novoseltsev VN, Arking R, Novoseltseva JA, Yashin AI. Evolutionary optimality applied to *Drosophila* experiments: hypothesis of constrained reproductive efficiency. Evolution 2002;56:1136–49.
22. Rose MR. Making SENSE: strategies for engineering negligible senescence evolutionarily. Rejuvenation Res 2008;11:527–34.
23. Rose MR, Drapeau MD, Yazdi PG, et al. Evolution of late-life mortality in *Drosophila melanogaster.* Evolution 2002;56:1982–91.
24. Finch CE. The biology of human longevity: inflammation, nutrition, and aging in the evolution of life spans. Burlington, MA: Academic, 2007.
25. Ideker T, Thorsson V, Ranish JA, et al. Integrated genomic and proteomic analyses of a systematically perturbed metabolic network. Science 2001;292:929–34.

26. Rudan I, Smolej-Narancic N, Campbell H, et al. Inbreeding and the genetic complexity of human hypertension. Genetics 2003;163:1011–21.
27. Goh K-I, Cusick ME, Valle D, Childs B, Vidal M, Barabasi A-L. The human disease network. Proc Natl Acad Sci U S A 2007;104:8685–90.
28. Cowley AW. The genetic dissection of essential hypertension. Nat Rev Genet 2006;7:829–40.
29. Weiss KM. Cryptic causation of human disease: reading between the (germ) lines. Trends Genet 2005;21:82–8.
30. Chen Y, Zhu J, Lum PY, et al. Variations in DNA elucidate molecular networks that cause disease. Nature 2008;452:429–35.
31. Emilsson V, Thorleifsson G, Zhang B, et al. Genetics of gene expression and its effect on disease. Nature 2008;452:423–8.
32. Sharpless NE, DePinho RA. How stem cells age and why this makes us grow old. Nat Rev Mol Biol 2007;8:703–13.
33. Funk WD, Wang CK, Shelton DN, Harley CB, Pagon GD, Hoeffler WK. Telomerase expression restores dermal integrity to in vitro-aged fibroblasts in a reconstituted skin model. Exp Cell Res 2000;258:270–8.
34. Torella D, Rota M, Nurzynska D, et al. Cardiac stem cell and myocyte aging, heart failure, and insulin-like growth factor-1 overexpression. Circ Res 2004;94:514–24.
35. Bronikowski AM, Carter PA, Morgan, et al. 2003. Lifelong voluntary exercise in the mouse prevents age-related alterations in gene expression in the heart. Physiol Genomics 2003;12:129–38.
36. Conboy IM, Conboy MJ, Wagers AJ, Girma ER, Weissman IL, Rando TA. Rejuvenation of aged progenitor cells by exposure to a young systemic environment. Nature 2005;433:760–4.
37. Kirkwood TB. Evolution of ageing. Nature 1977;270:301–4.
38. Arking R, Wells RA. Genetic alteration of normal aging processes is responsible for extended longevity in *Drosophila.* Dev Genet 1990;11:141–8.
39. Jones DM, Song X, Rockwood K. Operationalizing a frailty index from a standardized comprehensive geriatric assessment. J Am Geriatr Soc 2004;52:1929–33.
40. Klein BEK, Klein R, Knudtson MD, Lee KE. Frailty, morbidity and survival. Arch Gerontol Geriatr 2005;41:141–9.
41. Rahim NG, Harismendy O, Topol EJ, Frazer KA. Genetic determinants of phenotypic diversity in humans. Genome Biol 2008;9:215.1–.9.
42. Ruan H, Wu C-F. Social interaction-mediated life span extension of *Drosophila* CuZn superoxide dismutase mutants. Proc Natl Acad Sci U S A 2008;105:7506–10.

# Chapter 5
# Mild Stress and Life Extension in *Drosophila melanogaster*

**Éric Le Bourg**

**Abstract** Being subjected to a mild stress can increase resistance to a stronger stress, but the idea of using mild stress to improve aging has not been systematically assessed until recent years. Several studies in the fly *Drosophila melanogaster* have shown that various mild stresses (hypergravity, heat, cold, irradiation) increase longevity; some mild stresses also increase the resistance to strong stresses (e.g., heat) and delay behavioral aging. The synthesis of the 70 kDa heat shock protein can explain the resistance to heat but not the increased longevity. The increased longevity induced by hypergravity is, however, not explained by the synthesis of the antioxidant enzymes superoxide dismutase and catalase. Therefore, for the time being, no explanation exists for the increased longevity and the delayed behavioral aging induced by a mild stress.

**Keywords** Mild stress • hormesis • aging • longevity • stress resistance • behavioral aging • *Drosophila melanogaster*

**Abbreviations** CAT: Catalase; g: Gravity; HG: Hypergravity; Hsp: Heat shock protein; SOD: Superoxide dismutase

## 5.1 Introduction

Since the beginning of the last century, the average life span has increased from about 50 years to 75–85 years in developed countries, and functional decline has been postponed *(1)*. People often assume that one of the goals of our century of fast technological advances is to help people live still longer without suffering from the

É. Le Bourg
Université Paul-Sabatier Centre de Recherche sur la Cognition Animale,
UMR CNRS 5169, 31062 Toulouse cedex 9, France,
e-mail: lebourg@cict.fr

C. Sell et al. (eds.), *Life-Span Extension,* Aging Medicine,
DOI 10.1007/978-1-60327-507-1_5,

predicaments of old age. Researchers sharply debate the longevity limits of human beings *(2)*, and the possibility of increasing life span even more, but they all agree that helping people to have a more comfortable old age is of interest. The duty of biogerontologists, rather than simply increasing mean life span, is to find new ways to improve life during old age.

It is well known that being subjected to a mild stress can increase resistance to a stronger stress, the so-called acclimation response. For instance, exposure to 37°C increases survival at 40°C in *Drosophila melanogaster (3)*. However, the idea of using mild stress to improve aging has not been systematically assessed until recent years. It is expected that a mild stress could increase longevity, whereas a more severe stress obviously decreases it, in accordance with the hypothesis of hormesis, i.e., the beneficial effects of low doses of a stressful agent *(4)*. This article discusses the use of various mild stresses to increase longevity slightly, delay behavioral aging, and increase stress resistance, particularly in old age, in the fruit fly *D. melanogaster*. In the following, "longevity" is the mean life span of a group of flies.

## 5.2 Hypergravity

Hypergravity (HG), i.e., gravity levels higher than 1 g, the Earth gravity (g) level, is a stress because the animal subjected to a high g load has to adapt to a greater weight: a 3-g level means that the weight of the animal is magnified thrice. HG increases the metabolic demand of flies at the same rearing temperature, due to the higher weight, without the adverse consequences of increased temperatures in poikilotherms (increased speed of chemical reactions, decreased longevity, increased activity level). HG is obtained by putting flies in a continuously rotating centrifuge. In the following experiments, except when indicated, flies were subjected to HG for 2 weeks from the second day of adult life (except for stops twice a week to change the rearing vials) and then transferred to 1 g: These flies are called HG flies. Flies never subjected to HG are called 1 g flies. Except when indicated, the same temperature was used in the centrifuge and at 1 g (25°C); the gravity level was maintained at the 1- to 5-g range (1–7.38-g in some experiments); and flies were kept in groups of 15 virgin males or females.

### *5.2.1 Hypergravity Increases Longevity of Males*

HG males lived longer than 1-g males (Fig. 5.1, +10%–20%), but HG can have a negative effect on females. These results have been observed in two laboratories with two strains with differing mean longevity at 1 g. HG did not have a positive effect if flies spent a total of 12 days in HG with 4 days in HG followed by 3 days at 1 g, showing that males must be continuously exposed to HG to live longer. In contrast, 3 weeks of continuous exposure to HG increased the longevity of males

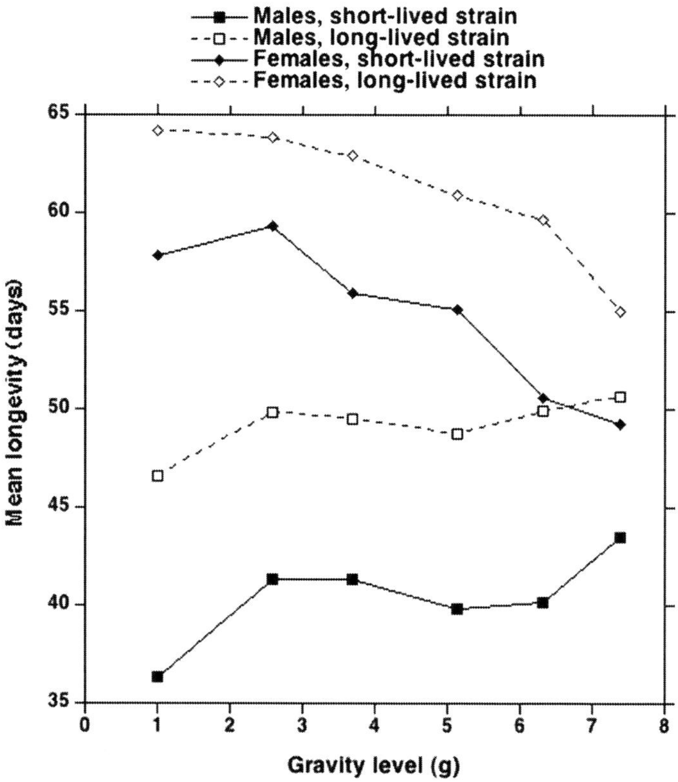


**Fig. 5.1** Effect of a 2-week stay in hypergravity, from the second day of adult life, on longevity. Two wild-type strains, differing in their mean longevity at 1 g, are used *(5)*. Each point is the mean of about 145 flies

but not 25 days. Three weeks in HG thus seems to be the limit between a mild stress with hormetic effect and a strong stress with no such effect, showing that the positive effect of HG can disappear if flies are subjected to a strong stress *(5–7)*.

It is possible, however, to modify the limit between a mild stress with positive effects and a strong stress with no such effect by improving or worsening the living conditions of flies. On the one hand, if males lived in individual vials after having spent 25 days in HG (individual rearing increases longevity), the long exposure to HG increased their longevity *(6)*. On the other hand, HG males kept continuously with females did not live longer than the 1-g males, probably because mating decreases longevity *(8)*. Similarly, if HG males were transferred at 28° or 30°C (which decreases longevity) after having lived in HG at 25°C, HG did not increase longevity *(8)*. Therefore, when flies are subjected to an extra stress with negative effects on longevity (mating and high temperature), the mild stress of HG can become a strong stress with negative effects on longevity. In contrast, subjecting flies to rearing conditions that increase longevity (individual rearing) produces the positive effects of long exposure to HG. In conclusion, HG has a hormetic effect on longevity.

### 5.2.2 Hypergravity Can Delay Behavioral Aging

Three behaviors that are affected by aging have been observed in HG flies. Climbing activity is the ability measured at the individual level to climb up the vertical side of a vial after having been subjected to a mechanical stimulus. The climbing score, which decreases with age, is the maximal height reached 20 s after the cessation of the mechanical stimulus. HG flies displayed a lower climbing score than 1-g flies the day following transfer to 1 g but higher scores some days later *(7, 9)*, all flies being unable to climb up at 5 weeks of age. This effect was mainly observed in males, but it could also be shown in females.

Young flies have straight paths when they are released at the center of an arena, whereas older ones have rather sinuous paths and do not move as far away from the center as young flies. Old HG flies moved further away from the center of the arena than 1-g flies, but HG had no effect on the sinuosity of the path *(9)*.

The spontaneous locomotor activity level, i.e., the number of motions recorded during a 12-h photophase, decreases with age. HG had no positive effect on spontaneous locomotor activity level in old age *(9)*.

These results show that, depending on the studied behavior, HG can delay behavioral aging or not.

### 5.2.3 Hypergravity Increases Resistance to Heat But Not to Other Stresses

A 1-, 2-, or 4-week exposure to HG starting the second day of life increased survival time at 37°C in both sexes (Fig. 5.2), but HG had no effect on resistance to cold (0°C) or desiccation, and decreased resistance to starvation *(5, 10, 11)*. To determine whether HG could also help flies recover from deleterious but nonlethal heat stress, such as a sudden but transient temperature rise, we simulated a summer heat wave by subjecting flies to 37°C for 60 or 90 min, which decreases longevity (–50%) after the heat shock but does not kill the flies during the shock. HG males heat-shocked at 4 weeks of age survived 15% longer than 1-g flies, but no positive effect of HG was observed at 5 or 6 weeks of age and in 4- to 6-week-old females. The heat shock decreased climbing activity and spontaneous locomotor activity scores, but HG did not counteract this effect at any age and in any sex. Therefore, HG protects against a deleterious nonlethal heat shock but not against the behavioral impairments due to this shock *(8)*. Flies were also subjected from 4 weeks of age to 4 heat shocks (30 or 45 min at 37°C) during a 2-week period. HG males lived 15% longer than 1-g flies, no effect being observed in females. Furthermore, living

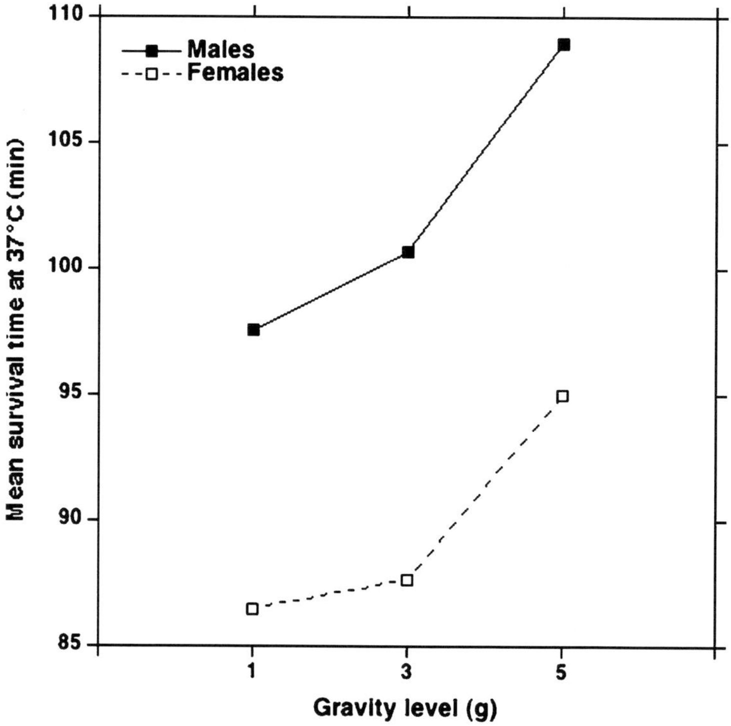


**Fig. 5.2** Effect of a 2-week stay in hypergravity, from the second day of adult life, on survival time at 37°C. Flies were placed at 2 weeks of age, after being transferred at 1 g, in tight vials in a water bath set at 37°C. The number of dead flies was recorded every 5 min up to the death of the last fly. Each point is the mean of about 45 flies *(7)*

in HG had nearly no effect on the difference in longevity between the HG and the 1-g groups when the deleterious effect of heat was moderate, i.e., when the longevity of the 1-g groups was not noticeably shortened by heat. In contrast, the difference in longevity between HG and 1-g groups was more important when heat shocks sharply decreased the longevity of 1-g flies *(12)*. In other words, males took advantage of a stay in HG if the negative effect of heat was important. Therefore, HG protects against a strong stress at middle age.

HG exposure did not confer any protection in either sex against oxidative stress. Flies were fed from the age of 19 days (i.e., 4 days after the end of centrifugation) an M/2 saccharose solution to which hydrogen peroxide (3.3% w/v) was added to decrease longevity; survival time was similar in all gravity groups. Another experiment used a 0.8% w/v hydrogen peroxide concentration at 16 or 27–28 days of age; HG had no positive effect on survival time *(13)*.

In conclusion, these results show that HG has hormetic effects on longevity, behavioral aging (but not on all studied behavioral traits), and resistance to heat (but not to other stresses). HG can thus help flies, particularly males, have a better old age.

## 5.3 Heat

### 5.3.1 *Heat Can Slightly Increase Longevity*

Heat has been used as a mild stress in several studies. The usual procedure is to subject flies to a single or repeated shocks at a high temperature (34–37°C) at a young age and to record their longevity.

A single heat shock (70 min at 36°C) slightly increased longevity by 2 days in virgin and mated flies ***(14)***. This modest effect was, however, more important in males (about 3 days) than in females (about 1 day), and the mean longevities were low in these experiments (i.e., between 23 and 40 days).

A similar longevity increase (1.5 day, sexes being not separated in longevity recording) was obtained in mated flies that were heat-shocked (100 min at 37°C) at 1 week of age, but no positive effect was observed in flies shocked at 4 weeks of age. The same heat shock applied at young, middle, or old age (9 weeks of age) decreased longevity of a more long-living strain ***(15)***.

Virgin and mated males and females of the inbred strain $w^{1118}$ lived longer (about 5 days) if subjected to a single, 20-min 36°C shock at 4 days of age, but heat shock had no effect or decreased longevity in transgenic flies overexpressing the 70 kDa heat shock-protein gene (*hsp70*) and in the control strain with no extra copies of the gene ***(16, 17)***.

Virgin flies of both sexes lived 2 days longer if subjected from 5 to 9 days of age to daily 5-min 37°C shocks, but longer daily shocks (10, 20, 40, 60 min) had no effect or decreased longevity ***(18)***.

Finally, mated females living in pairs or in groups of 10 females and 3 males that were subjected to a 3-h 34°C shock at 3, 6, 9, and 12 days of age lived 6 days longer than control flies. Decreasing the number of heat shocks made this positive effect disappear ***(19)***. The same procedure, but with only three shocks at 3, 6, and 9 days of age, had no effect on mutants harboring a heat-shock transcription factor inactivated at 30°C (this transcription factor is needed to synthesize heat shock proteins) or on females of a strain rescued by a functional *hsf* gene, but it increased by 4 days the longevity of males of this strain ***(20)***.

All of these results indicate that heat shock can increase longevity, even if the effect is modest, sometimes less than 2 days. They also show that that the window for a positive effect to be observed is narrow.

### 5.3.2 *Heat Does Not Clearly Delay Behavioral Aging*

Heat shock procedures that increased longevity (see above) had no positive effect on climbing activity ***(16, 18)*** and no effect on spontaneous locomotor activity measured throughout life in a wild-type strain ***(18)***. In contrast, heat shock increased spontaneous locomotor activity in the inbred strain $w^{1118}$, in transgenic flies overexpressing the 70 kDa heat shock-protein gene (*hsp70*), and in their control strain with no extra copies of the gene ***(16)***. Therefore, a positive effect of heat on behavioral aging is not clearly established.

### *5.3.3 Heat Increases Resistance to Some Stresses*

Pretreatment with heat increases resistance to a strong heat stress ***(14, 18–21)***, but in some cases this effect has not been observed ***(15)***. Otherwise, pretreatment with heat decreased starvation resistance but increased resistance to cold (10–15 min at −20°C) or to oxidative stress induced by paraquat in the inbred strain $w^{1118}$, in transgenic flies overexpressing the 70 kDa heat shock-protein gene (*hsp70*), and in their control strain with no extra copies of the gene ***(22)***. However, pretreatment with heat did not confer any protection in either sex against 0.8 or 3.3% w/v hydrogen peroxide in a wild-type strain ***(13)***.

In conclusion, these results show that heat has a slight hormetic effect on longevity, has no clear effect on behavioral aging, and increases resistance to some strong stresses.

## 5.4 Cold

### *5.4.1 Cold Increases Longevity*

Only two studies have used exposure to cold as a mild stress ***(13, 23)***. Exposing flies to 0°C for 1 h daily from 5 days of age for 2 periods of 5 days, separated by 2 days with no exposure, increased longevity by 10% (about 5 days). Depending on the experiment, the effect was significant in females or not ***(23)***. Survival time on saccharose, a poorly nutritious medium, was also increased by 2 days if flies were fed it after the last cold shock ***(13)***.

### *5.4.2 Cold Can Delay Behavioral Aging*

Flies exposed to the cold shock procedure that increased longevity (see above) had higher climbing scores than control flies (Fig. 5.3) ***(23)***. Therefore, cold has a positive effect on behavioral aging. Pretreatment with cold also decreased positive phototaxis in males but not in females ***(23)***.

### *5.4.3 Cold Increases Resistance to Some Stresses*

The cold shock procedure that increased longevity (see above) increased survival time at 37°C and percent of survival to a long cold shock (16 h at 0°C) in both sexes at 3, 4, 5, and 6 weeks of age, i.e., throughout life. In contrast, cold exposure

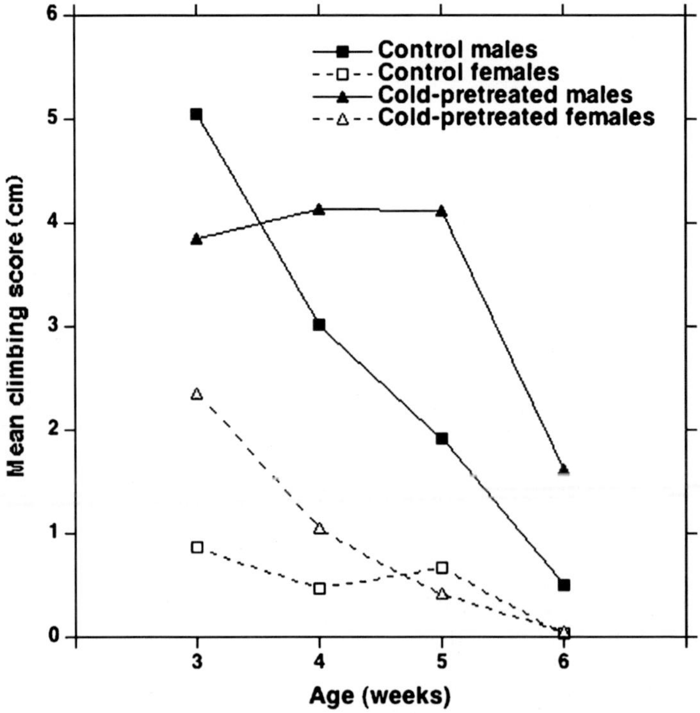


**Fig. 5.3** Effect of repeated exposure to cold on the mean climbing score. Flies were pretreated with cold or not (60 min daily at 0°C during two periods of 5 days separated by two days, starting at 5 days of age). The climbing score is the height (cm) reached by a fly in 20 s after the cessation of a mechanical stimulation. Each point is the mean of about 40 flies *(23)*

decreased survival time in flies that were starved. Flies were also subjected from 4 weeks of age to 4 heat shocks (30 or 45 min at 37°C) during a 2-week period. Flies exposed to cold lived about 15% longer after the first heat shock (about 2 days) than control flies if the heat shocks were 30-min long, but no effect of cold was observed with the 45-min heat shocks *(23)*.

Cold exposure provided a slight protection against oxidative stress in both sexes. Flies were fed from the age of 19 days (i.e., 3 days after the last cold shock) an M/2 saccharose solution to which 3.3% w/v hydrogen peroxide was added or not. Cold exposure increased survival time by less than half a day in the hydrogen peroxide group and by about 2 days in the saccharose groups. Other experiments were carried out at the same age with a different hydrogen peroxide concentration (0.8% w/v) or at 33 days of age with both 0.8% and 3.3% concentrations, and nonsignificant effects of cold exposure on survival time were observed. These experiments show that cold exposure has only a slight positive effect, if any, on resistance to hydrogen peroxide *(13)*.

## 5.5 Irradiation

An old controversy exists regarding the effects of low doses of irradiation on the longevity of *D. melanogaster*, because low doses have been reported either to increase or to decrease longevity or to have no effect ***(24)***. It has been argued ***(25)*** that low doses increase longevity only when flies live in poor rearing conditions, which could imply that any study showing a longevity increase is open to the criticism that inadequate rearing conditions were used. A similar problem occurred a few years ago when it was argued that overexpression of the Cu/Zn superoxide dismutase gene increased longevity only of short-lived strains ***(26)***. Obviously, showing a longevity increase in optimal living conditions is necessary to conclude that irradiation really increases longevity.

One issue with the old studies is that they usually did not record traits linked to the aging process, contrary to studies using high doses ***(27, 28)***. New results are summarized later.

### *5.5.1 Irradiation at the Egg Stage Increases Longevity*

As a hypothesis to explain longevity increases after low, repeated doses, it has been suggested ***(25)*** that irradiation kills bacteria and fungi in the vials containing flies. Even if it is not certain that bacteria and fungi decrease longevity ***(29, 30)***, one could overcome this problem by using irradiation at the egg or larval stage. Increased longevity has been observed in 9 out of 15 different genotypes irradiated with a total dose of 60 cGy during the entire preimaginal stage ***(31)***. If we disregard a wild-type strain, this study used mutants with a short life span. Increased longevity has also been observed in males of a wild-type strain irradiated with X-rays at the egg stage with a total dose of 0.5 and 0.75 Gy, but not with lower (0.25 Gy) or higher doses (1, 2, or 4 Gy) ***(32)***. No positive effect was observed in females (Fig. 5.4). The preadult viability of the irradiated eggs decreased slightly in the 0.25–1 Gy range (94% of viable eggs in the control group, 70% in the 1 Gy group), but more noticeably with the 2–4 Gy doses (respectively, 40 and 30%). In a later study, low doses also slightly increased longevity (Fig. 5.4) ***(33)***. Finally, irradiation of third-instar larvae with higher doses (1.2–17.1 Gy) decreased longevity ***(34)***.

### *5.5.2 Can Irradiation Delay Behavioral Aging?*

Unfortunately, no study has been done on this matter, but it is of interest to mention that flies irradiated at the egg stage with 0.25–1 Gy climbed up the sides of a vertical vial at 1 week of age faster than control flies ***(33)***. The same authors also observed that irradiated flies were faster to go to light, which is a form of locomotor activity

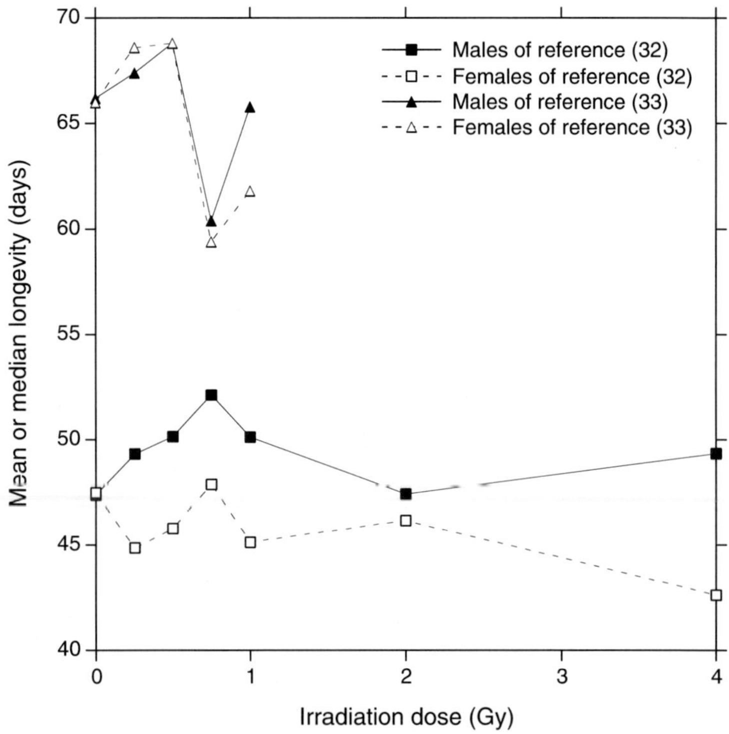


**Fig. 5.4** Effect of low doses of X-irradiation, in Grays, at the egg stage on adult longevity. The same strain was used in both studies. Each point is the mean of about 500 flies in ***(33)*** and the median of about 200 flies in ***(34)***

even if is not a perfect test of phototaxis (see ref. ***35*** for a discussion). It would be of interest to repeat these experiments throughout life rather than just at 1 week of age to determine whether irradiated flies age more slowly than control flies.

## *5.5.3 Irradiation Decreases Resistance to Heat and Desiccation*

In contrast to what has been observed with other mild stresses (see earlier), irradiation at the egg stage decreased the percent of survivors 24 h after a 90-min 38°C heat shock occurring at 1 week of age ***(33)***, whereas the same irradiation levels slightly increased longevity. The negative effect of irradiation was more evident in females than in males. Similarly, irradiation decreased resistance to desiccation ("dry starvation" in the article) in females irradiated with the lowest dose (0.25 Gy), whereas other doses had no effect. The authors only recorded the percent of survivors 18 h after beginning desiccation, which is a crude measure.

Paradoxically, the effects of low doses of irradiation on aging are still largely unknown, even if many studies have recorded the longevity of irradiated flies ***(24)***.

For the time being, it can be concluded that irradiation at the egg stage may slightly increase longevity and decrease resistance to stress. New studies on behavioral aging and resistance to stress in old age are needed.

## 5.6 What Are the Causes of Hormesis?

Previous sections of this chapter have shown that mild stresses can delay behavioral aging and increase longevity and resistance to some strong stresses. They can also decrease resistance to other stresses. These results tip the scales in favor of the positive effects of mild stresses, so discovering their causes is of interest. Most of the available research has been done using HG as a mild stress.

According to the well-known free radical theory of aging ***(36)***, aging is explained by the damage caused by free radicals produced during metabolism, despite the existence of antioxidant defenses. If this theory is correct, one would expect that increased activity of antioxidant enzymes could increase longevity: Are the effects of mild stress on longevity explained by increased activity of such enzymes? The activities of the antioxidant enzymes superoxide dismutase (SOD) and catalase (CAT) were measured at 2, 4, or 6 weeks of age in homogenates of individual HG flies and in 1-g flies: The gravity level had no effect on SOD and CAT activities at any age and in any sex ***(37)***. Therefore, flies that have lived in HG are not better protected from free radical attacks than those flies that always live at 1 g. Thus, the increased longevity of males is not linked to the increased activity of antioxidant enzymes, but other antioxidant defenses such as reduced glutathione have not been measured. The fact that mild stresses (heat, cold, and HG) do not confer resistance to hydrogen peroxide ***(13)*** seems to confirm the observation that mild stresses do not increase antioxidant defenses.

Heat shock proteins (Hsp) are molecular chaperones induced by various stresses in *D. melanogaster* and other species (reviewed in ref. ***38)***. The 70 kDa Hsp (Hsp70) is expressed, for instance, after a heat shock ***(21)***. Could increased production of Hsp70 explain the hormetic effects of HG? A Western immunoblot procedure showed that HG does not provoke Hsp70 synthesis but that more protein is synthesized after a heat shock (45 min at 37°C) in HG flies ***(7, 11)***. The HG-linked increased heat resistance could thus be explained by increased Hsp70 synthesis. The increased longevity or delayed behavioral aging of HG flies cannot be explained by Hsp70 because this protein is not synthesized at 25°C, the rearing temperature of flies. Because Hsp70 probably explains a part of the effect of HG, one may wonder whether transgenic flies overexpressing hsp70 would take advantage of more Hsp70 synthesis when subjected to HG. A study with a transgenic strain overexpressing hsp70 and a control strain with no extra copies of the gene showed that the positive effects of HG on survival time at 37°C are not increased in the transgenic strain and that no positive effect of HG on climbing activity at middle age or on longevity was observed in either the transgenic or the control strain ***(7)***.

The effects of HG on survival in response to heat, longevity, and behavioral aging are probably not due to a single cause: The increased resistance to heat is probably linked to the increased synthesis of Hsp70, whereas increased longevity and delayed behavioral aging are not explained by Hsp or by the antioxidant enzymes SOD and CAT.

It has also been shown that Hsp70 levels are increased in old females after a strong heat shock if the flies have been subjected to mild heat stresses at a young age ***(39)***. This result has been confirmed in flies, mainly males, of a strain harboring a heat shock transcription factor inactivated at 30°C (*hsf* gene) but rescued by a functional *hsf* gene ***(20)***. In contrast, flies of both sexes subjected to heat shocks at a young age, which slightly increased survival time at 37°C and longevity at 25°C, did not synthesize more Hsp70 after a 37°C heat shock than did control flies. These results were observed throughout life ***(18)***.

No other study of the mechanisms of mild stresses known to have hormetic effects has been done. Therefore, for the time being, it is impossible to explain the causes of hormetic effects.

## 5.7 Conclusions

It is well established that a mild stress can increase longevity, delay behavioral aging, and increase resistance to strong stresses in *D. melanogaster*. However, some stresses do not increase the longevity of females [e.g., (6)] or increase it only in some experiments ***(23)***. Similarly, the positive effects of mild stress on behavioral aging or resistance to a strong stress are often higher in males than in females ***(12, 23)***. The reason for these sex-linked differences remains obscure.

Positive effects of mild stress have been obtained in other species, such as the nematode *Caenorhabditis elegans* and rodents ***(40)***. The fact that mild stresses have positive effects in various species, even if studies of mammals are not still numerous, seems to indicate that there are "public" mechanisms modulating aging, that is, mechanisms shared across species, and that hormesis could be such a shared mechanism. Species have implemented a way to cope at a young age with mild stress that, as a side effect, has positive effects in old age, a time when most animals living in the wild are already dead ***(41)***. It is, however, premature to know whether mild stress will one day become a therapy for elderly people.

Mild stress increases the longevity of flies, but the increase is small, not exceeding 20%. Other authors have reported that diet restriction can also increase longevity in *D. melanogaster.* It would be of interest to compare the sizes of the effects induced by mild stress with those induced by diet restriction. Such a comparison is not easy to do because of the hot debate concerning the existence of an increase in longevity in flies subjected to diet restriction ***(42, 43)*** and the composition of the food regime that leads to increased longevity ***(44)***.

Other means to increase longevity in flies have been reported, such as chemicals ***(45)*** or mutations. For the time being, mild stress may be the only environmental means of increasing longevity and resistance to stress and delaying behavioral aging, even if these effects are not always of a large magnitude. The cause or causes of these beneficial effects of mild stress remain unknown.

## References

1. Robine JM, Michel JP. Looking forward to a general theory on population aging. J Gerontol Biol Sci 2004;59A:590–7.
2. Robine JM, Vaupel JW, Jeune B, Allard M, eds. Longevity: To the limits and beyond. Berlin: Springer, 1997.
3. Krebs RA, Loeschcke V. Effects of exposure to short-term heat stress on fitness components in *Drosophila melanogaster*. J Evol Biol 1994;7:39–49.
4. Calabrese EJ, Baldwin LA. Reevaluation of the fundamental dose-response relationship. Bioscience 1999;49:725–32.
5. Le Bourg E, Minois N, Bullens P, Baret P. A mild stress due to hypergravity exposure at young age increases longevity in *Drosophila melanogaster* males. Biogerontology 2000;1:145–55.
6. Le Bourg E, Minois N. Increased longevity and resistance to heat shock in *Drosophila melanogaster* flies exposed to hypergravity. C R Acad Sci III 1997;320:215–21.
7. Le Bourg E, Valenti P, Payre F. Lack of hypergravity-associated longevity extension in *Drosophila melanogaster* flies overexpressing hsp70. Biogerontology 2002;3:355–64.
8. Le Bourg E, Toffin E, Massé A. Male *Drosophila melanogaster* flies exposed to hypergravity at young age are protected against a non-lethal heat shock at middle age but not against behavioral impairments due to this shock. Biogerontology 2004;5:431–43.
9. Le Bourg E, Minois N. A mild stress, hypergravity exposure, postpones behavioral aging in *Drosophila melanogaster*. Exp Gerontol 1999;34:157–72.
10. Minois N, Le Bourg E. Resistance to stress as a function of age in *Drosophila melanogaster* living in hypergravity. Mech Ageing Dev 1999;109:53–64.
11. Minois N, Guinaudy MJ, Payre F, Le Bourg E. HSP70 induction may explain the long-lasting resistance to heat of *Drosophila melanogaster* having lived in hypergravity. Mech Ageing Dev 1999;109:65–77.
12. Le Bourg E. Hormetic protection of *Drosophila melanogaster* middle-aged male flies from heat stress by mildly stressing them at young age. Naturwissenschaften 2005;92:293–6.
13. Le Bourg E. Three mild stresses known to increase longevity in *Drosophila melanogaster* flies do not increase resistance to oxidative stress. Am J Pharmacol Toxicol 2008;3:137–43.
14. Khazaeli AA, Tatar M, Pletcher SD, Curtsinger JW. Heat-induced longevity extension in *Drosophila*. I. Heat treatment, mortality, and thermotolerance. J Gerontol Biol Sci 1997;52A:B48–B52.
15. Kuether K, Arking R. *Drosophila* selected for extended longevity are more sensitive to heat shock. Age 1999;22:175–80.
16. Minois N, Khazaeli AA, Curtsinger JW. Locomotor activty as a function of age and life span in *Drosophila melanogaster* overexpressing hsp70. Exp Gerontol 2001;36:1137–53.
17. Minois N, Vaynberg S. Fecundity and life span in transgenic *Drosophila melanogaster* overexpressing hsp70. Biogerontology 2002;3:301–6.
18. Le Bourg E, Valenti P, Lucchetta P, Payre F. Effects of mild heat shocks at young age on aging and longevity in *Drosophila melanogaster*. Biogerontology 2001;2:155–64.
19. Hercus MJ, Loeschcke V, Rattan SIS. Lifespan extension of *Drosophila melanogaster* through hormesis by repeated mild heat stress. Biogerontology 2003;4:149–56.
20. Sørensen JG, Kristensen TN, Kristensen KV, Loeschcke V. Sex specific effects of heat induced hormesis in Hsf-deficient *Drosophila melanogaster*. Exp Gerontol 2007;42:11239.
21. Dahlgaard J, Loeschcke V, Michalak P, Justesen J. Induced thermotolerance and associated expression of the heat-shock protein Hsp70 in adult *Drosophila melanogaster*. Funct Ecol 1998;12:786–93.
22. Minois N. Resistance to stress as a function of age in transgenic *Drosophila melanogaster* overexpressing hsp70. J Insect Physiol 2001;47:1007–12.
23. Le Bourg E. Positive effects of exposure to cold at young age on longevity, aging and resistance to heat or cold shocks in *Drosophila melanogaster*. Biogerontology 2007;8:431–44.
24. Lamb MJ. Radiation. In: Lints FA, Soliman MH, eds. *Drosophila* as a model organism for ageing studies. Glasgow: Blackie, 1988:71–84.

25. Sacher GA. Effects of X-rays on the survival of *Drosophila* imagoes. Physiol Zool 1963;36:295–311.
26. Orr WC, Sohal RS. Does overexpression of Cu/Zn-SOD extend life span in *Drosophila melanogaster*? Exp Gerontol 2003;38:227–30.
27. Miquel J, Lundgren PR, Binnard R. Negative geotaxis and mating behavior in control and gamma-irradiated *Drosophila*. Drosophila Information Service 1972;48:60–1.
28. Lamb MJ, McDonald RP. Heat tolerance changes with age in normal and irradiated *Drosophila melanogaster*. Exp Gerontol 1973;8:207–17.
29. Ren C, Webster P, Finkel SE, Tower J. Increased internal and external bacterial load during *Drosophila* aging without life-span trade-off. Cell Metab 2007;6:144–52.
30. Le Bourg E. Hormetic effects on longevity of hydrogen peroxide in *Drosophila melanogaster* flies living on a poorly nutritious medium. Biogerontology 2007;8:327–44.
31. Moskalev A. Radiation-induced life span alteration of *Drosophila* lines with genotype differences. Biogerontology 2007;8:499–504.
32. Vaiserman AM, Koshel NM, Litoshenko AY, Mozzukhina TG, Voitenko VP. Effects of X-irradiation in early ontogenesis on the longevity and amount of the S1 nuclease sensitive DNA sites in adult *Drosophila melanogaster*. Biogerontology 2003;4:9–14.
33. Vaiserman AM, Koshel NM, Mechova LV, Voitenko VP. Cross-life stage and cross-generational effects of gamma-irradiations on the egg stage of *Drosophila melanogaster* life histories. Biogerontology 2004;5:327–37.
34. Vaiserman AM, Koshel NM, Voitenko VP. Effect of X-irradiation at larval stage on adult lifespan in *Drosophila melanogaster*. Biogerontology 2004;5:49–54.
35. Le Bourg E, Badia J. Decline in photopositive tendencies with age in *Drosophila melanogaster* (Diptera: Drosophilidae). J Insect Behav 1995;8:835–45.
36. Harman D. Aging: A theory based on free radical and radiation chemistry. J Gerontol 1956;11:298–300.
37. Le Bourg E, Fournier D. Is lifespan extension accompanied by improved antioxidant defences? A study of superoxide dismutase and catalase in *Drosophila melanogaster* flies that lived in hypergravity at young age. Biogerontology 2004;5:261–6.
38. Morrow G, Tanguay RM. Heat shock proteins and aging in *Drosophila melanogaster*. Semin Cell Dev Biol 2003;14:291–9.
39. Kristensen TN, Sørensen JG, Loeschcke V. Mild heat stress at a young age in *Drosophila melanogaster* leads to increased Hsp70 synthesis after stress exposure later in life. J Genet 2003;82:89–94.
40. Le Bourg E, Rattan SIS, eds. Mild stress and healthy aging: Applying hormesis in aging research and interventions. Berlin: Springer, 2008.
41. Le Bourg E. Hypergravity in *Drosophila melanogaster*. In: Le Bourg E, Rattan SIS, eds. Mild stress and healthy aging: Applying hormesis in aging research and interventions. Berlin: Springer, 2008:43–63.
42. Le Bourg E, Minois N. Does dietary restriction really increase longevity in *Drosophila melanogaster*? Ageing Res Rev 2005;4:409–21.
43. Mockett RJ, Cooper TM, Orr WC, Sohal RS. Effects of caloric restriction are species-specific. Biogerontology 2006;7:157–60.
44. Vigne P, Frelin C. Diet dependent longevity and hypoxic tolerance of adult *Drosophila melanogaster*. Mech Ageing Dev 2007;401–6.
45. Massie HR. Chemicals. In: Lints FA, Soliman MH, eds. *Drosophila* as a model organism for ageing studies. Glasgow: Blackie, 1988:59–70.

# Part IV
# Rodents

# Chapter 6
# Global Food Restriction

**Michelle E. Matzko, Roger J. McCarter, and Edward J. Masoro**

**Abstract** The use of restricted feeding paradigms to understand mechanisms of aging in rodent models is discussed. The phrase *global food restriction* is defined so as to avoid ambiguities that have arisen with the use of the phrase *dietary restriction*. Evidence is evaluated regarding the claim that such procedures not only extend longevity but also retard aging processes. Several hypotheses that have been advanced to explain this action (such as growth retardation, reduction of body fat, decreased metabolic rate, decreased plasma levels of various metabolites, and decreased levels of oxidative damage) are assessed and found wanting. Evidence is described in support of an overall mechanism in which hormesis plays an important role. It is suggested that moderate reduction of energy intake constitutes a low-intensity stressor that results in the mobilization of cellular defense mechanisms. These defense mechanisms decrease the accumulation of the cellular molecular damage that underlies senescence. It seems likely that the energy-restricted animal now exists in a new metabolic state in which many, rather than few, metabolic characteristics are altered. Many or all of these altered metabolic characteristics may play a role in the beneficial effects of caloric restriction.

**Keywords** Caloric restriction • dietary restriction • extended longevity • mechanisms of aging • rodent models • hormesis

**Abbreviations** AGE: Advanced glycosylation end product; AL: Ad libitum; CR: Caloric restriction; DR: Dietary restriction; FOXO: Forkhead; GH: Growth hormone; IGF-I: Insulin-like growth factor I; MNCL: Mononuclear cell leukemia; MR: Metabolic rate; mtDNA: Mitochondrial DNA; NTG: Nontransgenic; PGC-1$\alpha$:

---

M.E. Matzko and R.J. McCarter (✉)
Center for Developmental and Health Genetics, The Pennsylvania State University, University Park, PA, 16802, USA
e-mail: rjm28@psu.edu

E.J. Masoro
Barshop Institute for Longevity and Aging Studies, University of Texas Health Science Center, San Antonio, TX, 78229, USA

C. Sell et al. (eds.), *Life-Span Extension,* Aging Medicine,
DOI 10.1007/978-1-60327-507-1_6,

Peroxisome proliferator-activated receptor coactivator 1; PPARα: Peroxisome proliferator-activated receptor alpha; RAGE: Receptor for advanced glycosylation end product; ROS: Reactive oxygen species; TG: Transgenic; TOR: Target of rapamycin

## 6.1 Overview

The use of dietary manipulations to modulate the aging phenotype has a long history, often with questionable claims of success. Both regimens that increase and those that decrease the intake of a dietary component, such as supplementing the diet with vitamin E or decreasing the dietary fat content, have been used. Moderately decreasing the food intake of rats and mice has been found to have markedly beneficial actions on the aging phenotype of these species. This dietary manipulation has been the subject of intense study and is often referred to as dietary restriction (DR), an unfortunate term because DR can also refer to a reduced intake of a specific nutrient. To avoid this ambiguity, *global food restriction* is used in this article instead of DR to denote this dietary regimen operationally. Both terms are replaced by *caloric restriction* (CR) when it is established that the responsible nutritional factor is a reduction in caloric intake.

### *6.1.1 Life Extension*

In 1935, McCay and colleagues *(1)* reported that restricting the food intake of rats after weaning resulted in a marked increase in longevity. Since then, many investigators have confirmed this finding in a spectrum of rat and mouse genotypes in studies that usually involved a 30–60% decrease in food intake *(2)*. Moreover, manipulations aimed at decreasing food intake have been reported to increase longevity of organisms in many other taxa *(3)* ranging from dogs, hamsters, and fish to flies, nematodes, spiders, and yeast. However, it remains to be established whether the mechanisms underlying life extension among these various taxa are the same or even similar. Rats and mice are the focus of this article.

Indeed, the question exists as to whether the mechanisms underlying global food restriction-induced life extension in mice are the same as those in rats. For example, global food restriction decreases the age-associated increased mortality rate of adult rats *(4, 5)*; in contrast, in some mice studies, global food restriction delays the age-associated increase in mortality rate but does not decrease the rate of increase once underway *(6)*. The magnitude of increase in mortality rate during adult life has long been viewed as an index of the rate of population aging *(7)*. Does this mean that global food restriction-induced life extension involves the slowing of the aging process in rats but not in mice? Or is this time-honored index of the rate of aging flawed? Driver *(8)* opts for the latter. Clearly, this is a conceptual issue that awaits resolution.

It should be further noted that the response of rats and mice to global food restriction differs in another regard. When it is initiated at advanced ages, global food restriction extends the life of mice ***(9)*** but not of rats ***(10)***.

### *6.1.2 Retardation of Physiological Deterioration*

In rodents as in other mammals, functional deterioration of physiological processes occurs with increasing age. Many of these functions have been found to remain in a youthful state at advanced ages in rats and mice on a long-term global food restriction regimen ***(11)***. However, two different life-span trajectories are responsible for this youthful state. In some of the processes, global food restriction attenuates the age-associated change; for example, it slows the age-associated increase in the level of serum cholesterol in rats ***(12)***. For other processes, global food restriction rapidly enhances the function but does not slow the subsequent age-associated change; for example, it enhances hepatic proteolytic capacity in young adult rats but does not affect the age-associated decrease in this process. This enhancement results in the hepatic proteolytic capacity of 24-month-old rats on a long-term global food restriction regimen being the same as that of ad libitum (AL)-fed 6-month-old rats ***(13)***. That global food restriction maintains physiological processes in a youthful state is often viewed as evidence of a slowing of the aging process. However, a caveat is in order: The use of physiological processes as biomarkers of the aging process is controversial ***(14)***.

### *6.1.3 Retardation of Age-Associated Diseases*

Global food restriction delays the occurrence and slows the progression of many different age-associated diseases in rats ***(15)*** and mice ***(16)***. This action includes many kinds of cancer ***(17)***, kidney disease ***(15)***, cardiovascular disease ***(18)***, neurodegenerative disease ***(19)***, autoimmune disease ***(20)***, cataracts ***(21)***, glaucoma ***(22)***, and osteoarthritis ***(23)***. It is tempting to believe that the retarding effect on such a broad range of diseases is due to the slowing of the aging process. However, again a caveat is in order: There is disagreement regarding what role, if any, the aging process plays in age-associated diseases ***(24)***.

## 6.2 Responsible Dietary Factor

In 1939, McCay et al. ***(25)*** reported that reducing caloric intake without reducing the intake of protein, vitamins, and minerals extended the life of rats; they concluded that the decreased intake of calories was the factor responsible for the life extension.

This conclusion was further supported some 50 years later by studies using semisynthetic diets, which permitted an assessment of the effect of the restriction of specific classes of dietary components on longevity. These studies showed that global dietary restriction-induced life extension is not due to the restriction of dietary protein ***(26)***, fat ***(27)***, minerals ***(27)***, or vitamins ***(28)***. By 1990, it was generally believed that the dietary factor responsible for the life-extending action of global food restriction was the decreased intake of calories, and the term CR was in general use when referring to this phenomenon.

However, this view was challenged by results from studies showing that markedly reducing the dietary intake of methionine significantly extended the life of rats ***(29)*** and mice ***(30)***. These findings gave rise to the speculation that reducing the intake of protein might be an important factor in global dietary restriction-induced life extension, which has led many to replace use of the term CR with DR. This speculation ignores the study of Masoro et al. ***(26)***, who showed that a 40% reduction in food intake without a reduction in protein intake is as effective in extending life as a 40% reduction in food intake with a 40% reduction in protein intake.

It should be noted that a marked reduction in methionine intake causes a severe imbalance in the intake of essential amino acids, which likely distorts metabolism and thereby stresses the animal. Thus, hormesis may well underlie the life extension resulting from the marked restriction of methionine intake by mice and rats. Hormesis is considered further below in regard to mechanisms responsible for the life-extending actions of CR.

## 6.3 Mechanisms Underlying Life Extension and Related Antiaging Actions

In more than 70 years since the seminal report of McCay and colleagues, many hypotheses have been put forth regarding mechanisms responsible for the effects of CR on longevity and the aging phenotype. None is strongly supported by the available evidence. The hypotheses that have had a major impact are discussed in this section, including evidence in support and against each hypothesis.

### *6.3.1 Growth Retardation Hypothesis*

In their 1935 paper ***(1)***, McCay and his colleagues proposed that reducing food intake increases longevity by retarding growth. This view prevailed among gerontologists until the 1980s, when studies were reported that showed that global food restriction initiated in adult mice ***(31)*** and rats ***(32)*** markedly extended their lives. In response to these two studies, most gerontologists abandoned the growth retardation hypothesis. However, recent information has led some to resurrect it. First, disrupting the growth hormone (GH)/insulin-like growth factor I (IGF-I) axis extends the life of mice *(33)*, and it is well known that CR lowers serum IGF-I levels *(34)*. Second, Miller et al. *(35)* reported that in a genetically heterogeneous mouse population, body weight from 2 to 24 months of age negatively correlated with longevity. In regard to this latter point, it should be noted that no correlation was found between body weight and longevity in the inbred F344 rat strain *(28)*. Thus, the finding of the Miller group is likely to have a genetic basis with little relevance to CR. Further information on the GH/IGF-I axis and its relationship to CR is presented in a later section of this chapter.

### *6.3.2 Reduced Body Fat Hypothesis*

In 1960, Berg and Simms *(36)* first proposed that the extension of life of rats on a long-term CR dietary regimen was due to a reduction in body fat content. However, in their study, body fat was not measured; rather these investigators assumed that the rats on a CR regimen must have a lower body fat content than the AL-fed rats. Their hypothesis was based on the emerging evidence some 50 years ago that a high body fat content adversely affected human health. Since then, many human studies have indicated a negative effect of high body fat content on human longevity. The Framingham Heart Study is an example of a well-controlled investigation strongly supporting this relationship *(37)*. The findings that mice with genetic obesity have a decreased longevity provided further support for this hypothesis *(38, 39)*.

It is important to note that neither of the genetic studies involved CR. Indeed, it was not until 1980 that the effects of CR on body fat content were reported by Bertrand et al. *(40)*. They found that CR markedly reduced total body fat as well as visceral fat of male F344 rats. Although the body fat content of the AL-fed group varied among the rats, no correlation was found between fat content and longevity in this group of rats. In the rats on the CR regimen, all of which were lean, a positive correlation was found between body fat content and longevity. Four years later, Harrison et al. *(41)* reported a study comparing obese *ob/ob* mice fed AL or caloric restricted with similarly treated lean mice that were congenic except for the *ob/ob* locus. They found the AL-fed *ob/ob* were shorter lived than the AL-fed lean mice but that the calorie-restricted *ob/ob* mice (48% adult body fat) were longer lived than the AL-fed lean mice (22% body fat). In fact, the calorie-restricted *ob/ob* mice were as long lived as the calorie-restricted lean mice (13% body fat). These two studies strongly indicated that the reduction in body fat content was not a major player in the life-extending action of CR and for some time there was little enthusiasm for the reduced body fat hypothesis.

In 1999, however, Barzilai and Gupta *(42)* resurrected the hypothesis based on the evidence that body fat, particularly visceral fat, secretes cytokines that have deleterious actions. Although not supported by empirical evidence, this concept stirred the imagination of many. In 2003, Blüher et al. *(43)* reported a provocative study on mice with a knockout of the insulin receptor specifically in the adipose tissue. The investigators called this animal model the FIRKO mouse. It has a

15–25% lower body weight and 50–70% less fat from 3 months of age on despite eating ~55% more food per gram body weight compared with nontransgenic mice. The mean life span of FIRKO mice was increased in both males and females by approximately 18%, median life span by 3.5 months, and maximum life span by ~5 months. In addition, leptin and plasma glucose levels were altered in unexpected ways. Leptin was ~25% higher in FIRKO mice than in controls ($p$ = NS), but when expressed as leptin per milligram of fat pad mass, leptin was ~3-fold higher in FIRKO mice ($p < 0.05$). Additionally, plasma glucose levels in FIRKO mice did not differ from those in the controls, and glucose tolerance was maintained throughout life compared with control mice, which had impaired tolerance at an advanced age ***(44)***. These findings are especially interesting with regard to leptin, which helps build the case for the importance of fat- and stomach-derived hormones (leptin, adiponectin, ghrelin) in metabolic processes. These hormones are increasingly implicated as important signalers of energy balance and are potential modulators of the relationship between CR and aging.

Although the findings of the FIRKO mouse studies are intriguing, the conclusion is not warranted that the effects of CR on longevity are due to leanness. First, CR was not studied. Second, the study does not establish that the life extension in the FIRKO mouse is due to the reduced fat mass. In addition to a reduction in fat mass, the FIRKO mouse has many metabolic differences compared with the wild-type mouse that have been described and likely many yet to be described. Indeed, no evidence was presented in support of a causal relation between the low fat mass and the life extension.

If the speculation is valid that a reduction in body fat is responsible for the CR-induced increase in life span, a reasonable expectation is that mice lacking white adipose tissue by genetic alteration might exhibit a longer life span. However, the opposite has been shown in several studies ***(45–47)***.

In summary, the evidence in support of the reduced body fat hypothesis is from investigations in which rodent life extension resulted from manipulations other than CR. The two studies that directly assessed the relationship between CR-induced life extension and body fat do not support the hypothesis. It seems likely, however, that reduction of body fat has some role in CR-induced life extension, but it clearly does not play a major role.

### *6.3.3 Decreased Metabolic Rate Hypothesis*

Few hypotheses of the mechanisms underlying life extension in CR have generated more controversy and been held as firmly as that of reduced metabolic rate (MR). The notion arises naturally from the fact that restricting food intake leads to a decrease in MR that is greater than can be accounted for on the basis of a change in body weight ***(48)***. As Garrow ***(49)*** has pointed out, "…there is no investigator who has looked for this effect and failed to find it." Sacher ***(50)*** coupled this fact with the rate of living theory of aging ***(51)*** to suggest that CR delays aging as a consequence of decreased energy metabolism, in accordance with the view that living tissues have a determined lifetime energy expenditure per unit mass. Additional support came from Harman's free radical theory of aging ***(52)*** because it was assumed that decreased rates of generation of damaging oxidative free radicals would accompany decreased rates of metabolism.

Data in support of this view include interspecific studies demonstrating increased longevity associated with decreased MR per unit mass (mass-specific MR) ***(53)*** and many reports of decreased MR in CR (for example, ***(49, 54–56)***) in animals ranging from mice to monkeys and humans. Additional support arises from documentation of reduced rates of generation of reactive oxygen species (ROS) ***(57, 58)*** in tissues of animals on long-term CR and decreased rates of oxygen consumption of mitochondria isolated from skeletal muscles of rats subjected to 12 months of CR, but not from those rats on CR for 18 months ***(59)***.

Evidence against this hypothesis is extensive and compelling: for example, CR rats (male, F344) that were allowed voluntary exercise ran 3–5 km/day over most of their life span. These animals had body weights significantly less than those of their sedentary CR counterparts and mass-specific MR significantly higher than that of sedentary CR animals and yet exhibited similar longevity, with increased 50% survival rate ***(60)***. Studies of food consumption and oxygen consumption over the life span of male F344 rats restricted by 40% in food intake ***(61, 62)*** demonstrated a transient decrease in a mass-specific MR (about 6 weeks' duration) followed by stabilization of MR over the remainder of life, so no significant decrease in MR occurred compared with that in control rats fed AL. Speakman et al. ***(63)*** and Selman et al. ***(64)*** found increased mass-specific MR in CR mice and in rats fed AL to be associated with increased longevity rather than decreased longevity. At the tissue and cellular levels, hepatocytes isolated from the livers of rats on CR for 4 months exhibited no significant differences in rates of oxygen consumption and ROS production from those isolated from control rats fed AL ***(65)***. Similarly, rates of resting oxygen consumption of skeletal muscles isolated from old F344 male rats (24–36 months old) were not different, whether from rats fed AL or fed 40% less than AL over the life span ***(66)***.

Although the preceding data suggest conflicting conclusions and controversy, the clear message is that decreased MR is neither necessary nor sufficient to explain life extension in CR; that is, decreased MR is not mechanistically involved in the action of CR on aging processes. Different effects have been observed in different animals, using different degrees of CR and different ages of initiation of restriction, but there is no consistent direction of change in MR in long-term CR. In the short term, there is no disagreement that mass-adjusted MR is decreased. In the long term, it seems clear that MR can remain decreased ***(67)***, be unaltered ***(62)***, or be increased ***(64)*** in animals with extended longevity. Similarly, discussions of the various normalization procedures are not pertinent to address the issue of applying rate of living criteria to mechanisms of action of CR, because the concept ***(51, 52)*** and its application to CR ***(50)*** are based on mass-adjusted values of MR. However, even if lowered MR in CR is examined in relation to individual tissues and organs, significant evidence remains against the hypothesis that CR acts by decreasing MR ***(63, 66)***. It should also be noted that consideration of large numbers of mammalian species identifies many species having both high MR and much greater longevity than would be predicted on the basis of the rate of living theory *(68)*. Whether or not altered rates of energy metabolism are mechanistically involved in aging processes, it seems clear that life extension by CR is not a consequence of reduced MR.

### 6.3.4 Oxidative Damage Attenuation Hypothesis

Oxidative damage to cellular components represents a balance between pro-oxidant factors (radicals generated by oxidative metabolism) and antioxidant processes (oxidative radical scavengers, repair and cellular turnover mechanisms). The demonstration in the early 1950s of the existence of reactive oxidative free radicals in situ *(69, 70)* led Harman *(52)* to propose that aging is a consequence of the inexorable accumulation of damage induced by oxidative radicals generated in the course of usual metabolism. The theory provided an immediate molecular basis for the rate of living theory of aging and has become widely accepted. Considerable experimental support comes from studies demonstrating the age-related accumulation of oxidative damage in tissues of a wide variety of species (reviewed in *(57)*) and from reports of age-related diseases in which oxidative damage plays a major role *(71)*. Whether or not the presence of increasing amounts of oxidatively modified molecules and cellular structures constitutes a mechanism of aging remains controversial *(72)*. For example, under- or overexpression *(73, 74)* of key antioxidant enzymes (MnSOD and CuZnSOD, respectively) has been demonstrated to lead to expected effects on tissue levels of oxidative damage but not to affect longevity in mice. In contrast, overexpression of a different antioxidant enzyme (catalase) was associated with extended survival in mice *(75)*. Moreover, naked mole-rats are similar in body size to mice but exhibit far greater longevity (25 years vs. 2 years, respectively), despite having greater levels (1.5- to 10-fold higher) of oxidative damage in various tissues at comparable fractions of the life span *(76)*.

Studies of the effects of CR provide additional support for this hypothesis. In general, CR is associated with reduced levels of oxidative damage, but the amount of reduction and the age at which decreased damage is detected in comparison with that in tissues of animals fed AL are variable. Many recent studies have focused on oxidative damage to lipids, proteins, and DNA of mitochondria. This focus is a consequence of the fact that most cellular oxidative free radical generation occurs in mitochondria, and, in the case of mitochondrial DNA (mtDNA), in particular, protection of the DNA molecules by associated histones is not present *(77)*.

Lipid peroxidation is considered an important index of oxidative damage because lipid peroxides and their decomposition products (such as aldehydes, ketones, epoxides) may affect the structure and function of cell membranes, both plasma membranes, and those of organelles such as mitochondria. Early studies demonstrated decreased accumulations with age of lipofucsin, malondialdehyde, and other lipid peroxides in brain and liver tissues of mice on CR diets *(78–80)*. Extensive studies by Yu and colleagues demonstrated decreased lipid peroxidation of hepatocytes and T lymphocytes isolated from rats on CR diets and identified a modification of lipid composition induced by CR (lower unsaturation/saturation index) rendering the associated membranes less susceptible to peroxidation and preserving their fluidity ***(80, 81)***. A great deal of more recent research has confirmed and extended these important initial observations ***(82)***.

Protein oxidation is similarly decreased by CR diets, but great diversity exists in reported findings for different tissues and even within a given tissue. For example, whole brain tissue in mice exhibits a 35% lower protein carbonyl (marker of protein oxidative damage) content for animals on a 40% restricted feeding diet in comparison with mice fed AL. However, the carbonyl content of the hippocampus was little affected by CR whereas the striatum exhibited a decrease of 48% in protein carbonyl content in the same animals ***(83)***. The carbonyl content of mitochondrial proteins isolated from hind-limb muscles of mice fed AL increased by 150% between ages 12 and 29 months whereas similar mice fed 40% less food exhibited no change in mitochondrial carbonyl content over the same age range ***(84)***.

Oxidative damage to DNA occurs in several different forms, such as single- and double-strand breaks, point mutations, and cross-links. One frequently used marker of oxidatively damaged DNA, derived from the interaction of DNA and the hydroxyl radical, is 8-OHdG (hydroxyl-2′-deoxyguanosine). Kaneko et al. ***(85)*** demonstrated increased concentration of this marker for nuclear DNA in kidneys of 24-month-old mice and in nuclear DNA from the hearts and livers of mice aged 27 months. However, for mice on a CR diet, these increases occurred only after 30 months of age. CR diets have also been effective in slowing the age-related accumulation of oxidatively damaged mtDNA, as measured by deletion frequency in livers from male rats ***(86)***. However, the effect of the CR diet was only manifested after middle age (rats 18 months and older) and was not found for mtDNA extracted from the brains of these rats.

The preceding examples represent a small sample from the extensive literature documenting the effectiveness of the CR regimen in reducing the rates at which oxidatively modified lipids, proteins, nuclear DNA, and mtDNA accumulate in different tissues. Although relatively few markers of oxidative damage have been used to assess effects in lipids, proteins, and nucleic acids, there is little question that CR exerts a powerful protective effect against oxidative damage in various tissues ***(87, 88)***.

Despite general agreement regarding the beneficial effects of CR on the attenuation of age-related oxidative damage, no causal link between such damage and mechanisms of aging has been established. For example, animals having altered levels of oxidative damage in various tissues nevertheless did not exhibit altered longevity ***(73, 74)*** nor did they exhibit longer survival in comparison with animals having lower levels of tissue oxidative damage ***(76)***. These effects of CR therefore may or may not play a role in retarding aging processes. Much work remains to be done in this important area. Merry ***(88)*** pointed out, “The generic conclusion that CR feeding regimes retard the accumulation of oxidative damage represents an over simplification resulting from gross tissue averaging.” As described previously, marked diversity of oxidative damage exists in response to both age and CR within and between tissues. Also, characteristic features of the effect of CR on aging, such as dose–response relationships between survival and degree of CR (and the duration of CR), have not been demonstrated with respect to the oxidative damage attenuation hypothesis. Do similar dose–response relationships exist between CR and oxidative damage? Given these uncertainties and difficulties, the significance of the effect of CR in attenuating age-related accumulation of oxidative damage remains unclear.

### *6.3.5 Decreased Glycemia Hypothesis*

An important characteristic of CR is that most tissues are affected by it. This intriguing finding suggests that, whatever may be its mechanism of action, it probably involves processes shared by most cells. In this regard, glucose constitutes a viable candidate because of its role as a primary source of fuel for all tissues, from red cells of blood to neurons of the brain and fibers of skeletal muscles. Levels of circulating glucose are closely regulated to similar values in different mammalian species and much evidence supports its essential role in the maintenance of homeostasis and health of the individual. Discussion is ongoing of the possibility that glucose may play a role in mechanisms of aging in general and in mechanisms by which CR modulates aging in particular ***(89, 90)***.

The connection between CR and glucose arises from the finding that animals on CR exhibit consistently lower levels of average daily plasma glucose – about 15 mg/dl, or 12% less in male F344 rats on long-term CR ***(91)***. Despite lower daily levels of circulating glucose and insulin, however, these rats on CR exhibit the same rates of utilization of glucose and the same levels of carbohydrate intake per unit of body mass ***(61, 62)***. Animals on CR therefore maintain appropriate daily fluxes of this important fuel but under conditions of lower circulating levels of glucose. The decreased daily level of plasma glucose has potential importance for mechanisms of action of CR, because glucose can undergo nonenzymatic reactions with amino groups of proteins and nucleic acids, thereby modifying their structure and function. This so-called Maillard reaction involves several stages in which a reducing sugar reacts with an amino group to form first a Schiff base, followed by a slow rearrangement to form an Amadori product. These reactions are reversible. With time, however, the Amadori product can undergo further transformations to yield an advanced glycosylation end product (AGE) ***(92)***, which is highly reactive and potentially damaging. Formation of AGE compounds is not limited to extracellular structures, because intracellular fructose and other phosphorylated sugars are far more potent glycating agents than is glucose ***(93)***. More recent research has identified potential mechanisms of tissue injury by AGEs: up-regulation of inflammatory processes via the binding of AGEs to cell surface receptors or RAGEs ***(94)***. In addition, AGE compounds promote oxidative stress through the formation of ROS and vice versa, so that AGEs and ROS exert a positive feedback in the generation of compounds that are capable of creating the exponentially increasing degeneration of tissue structure and function characteristic of aging processes ***(95)***. Consistent with this notion, rates of formation of AGE compounds in tissues of various mammalian species have been found to be inversely related to longevity on a logarithmic scale ***(93)***. Finally, as noted by Cerami in his proposed model of "glucose as a mediator of aging" ***(89)***, several of the adverse consequences of chronic diabetes mellitus are similar to those of aging, such as atherosclerosis, cataracts, and impaired immune function. It seems clear, therefore, that elevated levels of circulating glucose and increased levels of AGE compounds are associated with tissue degeneration and impaired function as found with advancing age. The issue then is whether or not reduced levels of plasma glucose, as in CR, are mechanistically involved in the actions by which CR retards aging processes.

A recent test of this hypothesis ***(96)*** was made possible by the availability of genetically manipulated, transgenic mice having levels of plasma glucose under fully fed conditions similar to those of nontransgenic littermates fed a CR diet (40% less food than control mice fed AL). Two groups of male mice [nontransgenic (NTG) C57BL/6; transgenic (TG) overexpressing a human GLUT4 minigene in fat, cardiac, and skeletal muscle tissues on a C57BL/6 background] were fed either AL (NTGA, TGA) or 40% less than AL (NTGR, TGR) from 6 weeks of age onward. It should be noted that daily food consumption, as well as body weights, was the same for both transgenic and nontransgenic mice. Average daily levels of plasma glucose were highest in NTGA mice, lowest in TGR mice, and in-between for NTGR and TGA mice that had similar plasma glucose levels. Differences in plasma glucose levels were sustained over the life span, resulting in three different levels of average daily glycemia in the four different groups of mice. Longevity, physiological characteristics, and tissue damage were measured. Results were unambiguous: survival, function, and tissue damage were characterized by levels of food intake and not by levels of plasma glucose. The authors concluded that decreased plasma glucose over the life span is not an important factor in CR-induced life extension.

## 6.3.6 *Insulin Hypotheses*

In 1992, Masoro et al. ***(97)*** reported that rats on a long-term CR regimen maintained mean 24-h plasma glucose and insulin concentrations significantly lower than rats fed AL. They also found that the daily use of glucose as a fuel occurred at the same rate in rats on the CR regimen as in AL-fed rats when the data are expressed per kilogram body weight to the three-quarter power and concluded that CR either enhanced glucose effectiveness or increased insulin sensitivity as defined by Bergman ***(98)***. In contrast, Kenyon et al. ***(99)*** reported in 1993 that a loss of function mutation in the insulin-like signaling system of *Caenorhabditis elegans* markedly extended life; subsequently, similar findings were reported for *Drosophila melanogaster* ***(100, 101)***.

### 6.3.6.1 Increased Insulin Sensitivity Hypothesis

In 2000, Gupta et al. ***(102)*** showed that rats on a CR regimen do indeed exhibit increased insulin sensitivity. Does the increased insulin sensitivity play a role in CR's life-extending and related actions? Although this question has not been definitively answered, some empirical evidence supports this hypothesis ***(33)***.

#### 6.3.6.2 Decreased Insulin Signaling Hypothesis

The study of Blüher et al. ***(43)*** provides support for this hypothesis. They found that mice with the insulin receptor specifically disrupted in the adipose tissue (designated the FIRKO mouse) exhibited a 14% increase in maximal life span. It should be noted that the procedure used for the generation of the FIRKO mouse is not totally specific in targeting only adipocytes; it also disrupts macrophage insulin receptors ***(103)***. Within the context of CR, the increased life span of the FIRKO mouse is both a provocative and somewhat puzzling finding in that CR-induced life extension is associated with enhanced insulin sensitivity. By 10 months of age, however, the FIRKO mouse also exhibits increased insulin sensitivity compared with the wild type despite the disruption of the adipose tissue insulin receptor ***(44)***. It is also important to note that complete or heterozygous disruption of the insulin receptors in liver or skeletal muscle results in insulin resistance with an increased risk of morbidity and mortality ***(104)***. The recent report of Taguchi et al. ***(105)*** provides further support for the decreased insulin-signaling hypothesis; they engineered mice with a reduced level of brain insulin receptor substrate 2 and found that these mice have an increased life span along with an increase in insulin resistance ***(105)***.

#### 6.3.6.3 Reconciling the Two Hypotheses

At first glance, it would seem that these two insulin hypotheses are mutually exclusive. Further consideration, however, suggests that they may operate in tandem in the following way: CR increases insulin sensitivity in the major sites of glucose fuel use such as skeletal muscle. Indeed, empirical evidence shows that it has such an action in skeletal muscle ***(106)***. This action enables glucose fuel use to be maintained along with reduced insulin levels. The reduction in insulin levels decreases insulin signaling in adipose tissue in brain regions as well as in other possible sites; this action in turn slows the aging processes and extends life by altering the secretion of humoral factors by adipocytes and macrophages such as the enhanced secretion of adiponectin ***(44)*** and by influencing neural functions of specific brain sites. Although this speculation is compatible with the currently available experimental findings, further empirical information is clearly needed to establish it as fact rather than fancy.

### *6.3.7 The Growth Hormone/Insulin-Like Growth Factor I Hypothesis*

Substantial evidence exists to support the idea that changes in the GH/IGF-I axis, long known as the major effector of mammalian growth and development, occur with advancing age. Declines in levels of plasma GH and IGF-I with age have been well characterized, and impaired GH secretion in response to various stimuli has been documented in older men and women ***(107–109)***. Studies indicate that a loss in diurnal pulses of GH secretion, together with an impairment in the ability of GH to induce IGF-I gene expression, contributes to decreased plasma IGF-I levels in both aging humans ***(110)*** and rodents ***(111, 112)***. Indeed, by the end of the twentieth century, it was generally believed that reduced levels of GH/IGF-I were a cause of senescent deterioration, and this led to therapeutic treatment of the elderly with GH supplements.

However, studies in various model systems suggest a contrary hypothesis, namely that reduced activity of the GH/IGF-I axis may be associated with extended longevity and decreased rate of aging. Experimental support for this hypothesis comes from Holzenberger et al. ***(113)***, who demonstrated that male and female mice that expressed only one copy of the *Igf1r* (Igf-I type I receptor) gene ($Igf1r^{+/-}$) lived on average 26% longer than homozygous *Igf1r*-expressing ($Igf1r^{+/+}$) littermates ($p < 0.02$). Sex differences regarding longevity were apparent: female heterozygous knockouts lived 33% longer than control females ($p < 0.001$), but differences among males were not significant. Other models that have implicated GH and IGF-I in the aging process are the Laron, Snell, and Ames dwarf mice. All three models have loss of function mutations at specific sites along the GH/IGF-I axis and all have shown increases in life span vs. genetically intact sibling controls. Both male and female Laron dwarf mice, which are homozygous for loss of the GH/receptor binding protein gene, demonstrate a life span extended by nearly 1 year ($p < 0.0002$) ***(114)***. In a seminal work, Flurkey et al. ***(115)*** reported a significant extension of life span in Snell dwarf mice, characterized by an underdeveloped pituitary and therefore low GH and IGF-I. Due to small sample size, separate analyses of males and of females could not confirm a significantly longer life span in dwarf mice, but taken together data showed that male and female dwarf animals had significantly longer life spans than sibling controls (1,178 ± 235 days for dwarf animals vs. 832 ± 158 days for controls; $p < 0.001$). This difference represents a 42% increase in life span. Ames dwarf mice also display a nearly 50% extension of life span with their GH/IGF-I axis mutation ***(116)***. However, this specific model involves many coexisting endocrine disruptions caused by the general loss of pituitary function.

What evidence is there that low levels of GH/IGF-I may be involved in the life-extending effects of CR? Support emerges from the work of Bonkowski et al. ***(33)***. Male and female GHRKO mice (with a targeted loss of GH receptor binding protein) and their genetically intact siblings ($^{+/+}$) were subjected to 30% CR or fed AL. Wild-type ($^{+/+}$) mice undergoing 30% CR demonstrated the expected benefits of long-term CR. Male and female mice on the CR regimen had decreased body weight and increased average, median, and maximum life span. GHRKO mice subjected to CR also had reductions in body weight, but there was no effect of CR on average or median life span for either male or female GHRKO mice. Maximal life span extension in female ($^{+/+}$) mice undergoing CR was 19% compared with that in AL controls ($p < 0.05$), but the effects of CR on female GHRKO mice only increased maximum life span by 9% ($p < 0.05$). GHRKO mice on an AL diet had significantly improved insulin sensitivity compared with ($^{+/+}$) controls, and insulin sensitivity was not further improved by CR in male or female GHRKOs. These results are persuasive, suggesting that CR has little effect on longevity or insulin sensitivity in animals with diminished GH receptor and binding proteins, although the sexual dimorphism must be further explored. Moreover, Hursting et al. ***(117)*** presented findings showing that low levels of GH and IGF-I may play a role in the tumor-suppressive effects of CR. Rats subjected to 25% CR had serum levels of GH and IGF-I more than 50% lower than AL controls and greater inhibition of mononuclear cell leukemia (MNCL, a malignant neoplasm) proliferation in situ, latency to spread, and severity. Restoring GH and IGF-I levels in CR rats increased MNCL proliferation to the level seen in AL rats. A subsequent in vitro model showed that cultured MNCL cells proliferated less in the presence of serum from CR animals than in that from AL animals. This report provides additional evidence that low levels of GH and IGF-I may be involved in mechanisms by which CR carries out its anticarcinogenic effects. Taken together, the studies suggest that maintenance of signaling in the presence of reduced levels of GH and IGF-I may form part of the mechanism by which CR delays aging and its morbidities. Consistent with this view, Sonntag et al. ***(118–120)*** have postulated that IGF-I is a key player in the relationship between CR and the increased protein synthesis observed in restricted animals. The authors found that IGF-I was approximately 40% lower in young CR animals vs. AL-fed animals, and the CR animals exhibited no age-related decline in IGF-I as is found in AL-fed animals. However, the authors also determined that IGF-I receptors are 1.5- to 2.5-fold upregulated in heart, liver, and skeletal muscle in old CR animals but not in old AL animals and that CR animals exhibited normal GH pulsatility, which was lost during aging in AL animals. These data therefore suggest that CR enables the maintenance of a youthful phenotype (GH pulsatility, signaling) despite lower levels of IGF-I.

Overall, it seems possible that reduced activity of the GH/IGF-I axis may be involved in the antiaging actions of CR. However, the importance of alterations in the GH/IGF-I axis for the life-extending action of CR remains an unanswered question.

## *6.3.8 The Hormesis Hypothesis*

Most of the many proposed hypotheses regarding the biological mechanism(s) underlying CR-induced life extension are based on processes that CR is known to affect. It is indeed likely that many of these play some role in its life-extending action. The scope of each is, however, too narrow to provide a fundamental understanding of the antiaging actions of CR. The hormesis hypothesis may provide the framework needed for a full understanding. Masoro ***(121)*** and Turturro et al. ***(122)*** independently proposed this hypothesis in 1998.

### 6.3.8.1 Hormesis: Definitions and Concepts

Hormesis is broadly defined as the qualitative difference in the response of organisms when they are exposed to a physical or chemical agent at high intensity compared to exposure at low intensity ***(123)***. For example, continuous high doses of gamma rays decrease the life span of mice whereas low doses increase their life span *(124)*. Toxicologists use hormesis to refer to the beneficial effect of chemical agents at low concentrations that are toxic at higher concentrations *(125)*. For use within the context of biological gerontology, Rattan *(126)* has refined the definition of hormesis as follows: Hormesis in aging is characterized by the beneficial effects resulting from the cellular responses to mild repeated stress.

#### 6.3.8.2 Caloric Restriction, A Low-Intensity Stressor

Elevation of the plasma level of glucocorticoids is recognized as a signature response of mammals to stressors *(127)*. Sabatino et al. *(128)* studied the circadian rhythm in rats of plasma-free corticosterone concentration and found the daily peak concentration to be modestly but significantly elevated in those on a CR regimen compared to AL-fed animals. They further reported that the elevation in the level of free corticosterone in plasma in response to CR was small in comparison to that caused by a brief restraint stress. These findings strongly indicated that CR acts as a daily low-intensity stressor throughout most of the life of the animals in long-term studies.

#### 6.3.8.3 Caloric Restriction, A Hormetic Agent

If CR acts as a hormetic agent in rats and mice, it should enhance their ability to cope with intense stressors. There is evidence that it does so. In both young and old rats, CR decreases the short-term loss of body weight in response to surgery *(121)*. In young mice, it attenuates the inflammatory response following the injection of an inflammatory agent into the footpad *(129)*. In rats, it increases their ability to survive a sudden marked increase in environmental temperature *(130)*. CR also protects mice and rats against the harmful effects of a spectrum of toxic chemicals *(131, 132)*.

Thus, CR fulfills the classic criteria for a hormetic agent. A moderate reduction in energy intake protects against harmful agents, extends life, and retards aging processes, whereas a more severe reduction in energy intake is harmful, indeed lethal if the reduction is sufficiently marked.

#### 6.3.8.4 Relevance of the Hormetic Action of Caloric Restriction to Life Extension and Aging

Within the context of gerontology, aging is defined as the progressive deterioration of organisms throughout much of their adult life; that is, aging and senescence are synonyms. It is generally believed that this deterioration results from molecular damage from both endogenous (e.g., generation of reactive oxygen molecules during fuel use) and exogenous (e.g., environmental toxic chemicals) agents. Based on this view, the rate of aging is determined by the extent to which the damaging processes are not balanced by protective (e.g., antioxidant activities) and repair (e.g., DNA repair) processes. The rates of aging and longevity correlate negatively, and most biological gerontologists believe that CR extends life by slowing the rate of aging.

Rattan ***(133)*** has proposed that hormesis retards aging and extends life by augmenting protective and repair processes. Indeed, many low-intensity stressors other than CR have been found to extend the lives of invertebrate species ***(134)***. Moreover, genetic manipulations in nonmammalian species that extend life are often found also to increase resistance to harmful stressors ***(135)***.

Thus, there is strong evidence that hormesis plays an important role in the antiaging and life-extending actions of CR. What is missing is knowledge regarding the nature of the signals and the pathways linking these signals to the repair and protective cellular processes. Section 6.4 summarizes what is currently known regarding signaling processes in the actions of CR, including those potentially involved in hormetic signaling.

## 6.4 Conclusions: Synthesis of Current Knowledge

In this synthesis, use is made of the lifetime data on body mass, food intake, and energy balance of male F344 rats either fed AL or restricted to 60% of the food intake of the AL-fed rats starting at 6 weeks of age ***(28, 32, 61)***. CR markedly increased the median and maximum length of life of these rats. This section is based on the assumption that common mechanisms underlie the life-extending action of CR in both genders of all rat and mouse strains. Figure 6.1 is a schematic summary of the current status of knowledge of potential processes involved in the longevity-promoting and related actions of CR in these rodent species. The text below is a verbal expansion of this schematic summary.

During the first 6 weeks on the CR regimen, the energy intake per gram of body weight of the male F344 rats on the CR diet was lower than that of the AL-fed control rats of the same age ***(61)***. Plasma levels of important hormonal and metabolic substances also differed between these two dietary groups. During this time, the rats on the CR regimen had lower concentrations of plasma glucose ***(97)***, insulin ***(97)***, IGF-I ***(136)***, and $T_3$ ***(137)*** and higher concentrations of plasma free corticosterone ***(138)***. It is also likely that the rats on the CR regimen exhibit decreased target of rapamycin (TOR) signaling, but supporting empirical evidence is as yet lacking. These changes in plasma levels are likely part of a nutrient deprivation response or stress response or more likely a result of both. Although both the nutrient deprivation and the stress responses have much in common, they probably differ in some specifics.

After the rats were on the CR regimen for 6 weeks, the intake of food per gram of body weight of the restricted F344 rats reached and then exceeded that of the AL-fed rats of the same age ***(61)***. Indeed, over most of the remaining life of the AL-fed rats, both rat groups had the same daily food intake when normalized for lean body mass ***(61)***. Moreover, for most of their life span, the CR rats were in a positive energy balance ***(28)***. Thus, after 12 weeks of age, it seems unlikely that the

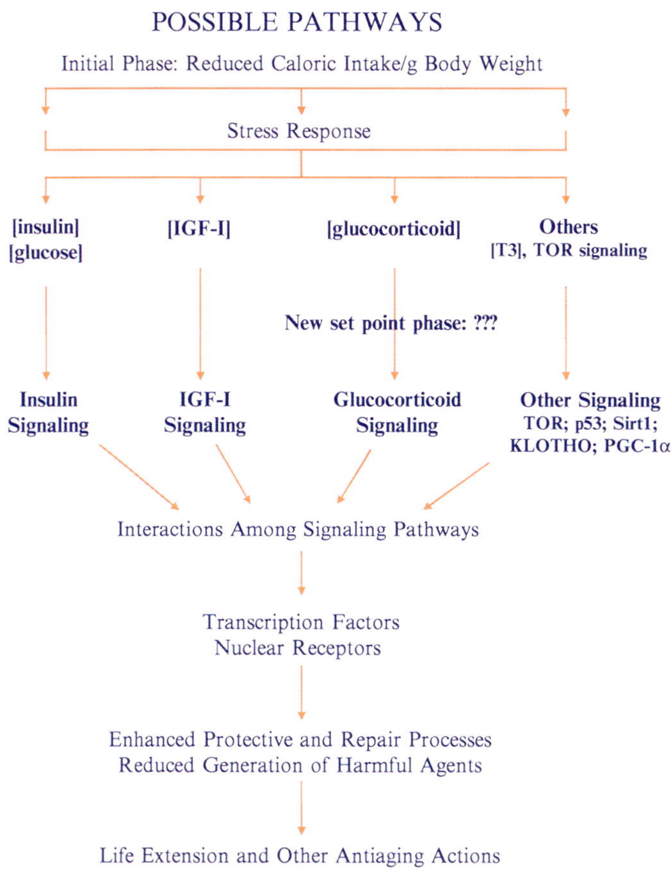


**Fig. 6.1** Possible signaling pathways linking caloric restriction to its life-prolonging and antiaging actions. *IGF-I* insulin-like growth factor I, *PGC-1α* peroxisome proliferator-activated receptor coactivator 1, and *TOR* target of rapamycin

rats on the CR regimen were experiencing either a nutrient deprivation response or a stress response.

This observation presents a dilemma because occurrences after 12 weeks of age were found to play the major role in CR-induced life extension of these F344 rats *(32)*. The fact that the rats on the CR regimen continued to have reduced levels of plasma glucose *(97)*, insulin *(97)*, IGF-I *(117, 139)*, and $T_3$ *(140)* and elevated levels of plasma free corticosterone *(138)* adds to the conundrum. Richardson and McCarter *(141)* suggested that a new homeostatic set point is established during the CR-induced period of nutrient deprivation and moderate stress and lasts for most of the remainder of the life span.

Expanding on this concept, we propose that the sustained alterations of the plasma hormone and metabolite levels are part of this new homeostatic set point and play a major role in the life extension. Indeed, the reduction in plasma levels of insulin and IGF-I probably decreases their signaling at key anatomic sites. As discussed in Sect. 6.3, this decreased insulin and IGF-I signaling slows the aging processes and extends the life. In addition, the elevated level of plasma-free glucocorticoid is known to enhance the ability to cope with damaging agents ***(127)***, and extension of life span is frequently associated with an increased resistance to damage ***(142)***. Viewing the regulatory signaling pathways involved in the life-prolonging and antiaging actions of CR solely in terms of insulin, IGF-I, and glucocorticoids is, however, too simple. There is evidence for the involvement of other pathways that act independently of as well as interactively with the IGF-I and insulin signaling pathways. The following such pathways or components of such pathways have been implicated: TOR ***(143)***, sirtuin proteins ***(144)***, peroxisome proliferator-activated receptor coactivator 1 (PGC-1$\alpha$) ***(145)***, p53 ***(146)***, and Klotho ***(147)***. In the case of each of these, however, much more must be done to be certain that it plays a role and, if so, to determine exactly what that role is. Moreover, it is likely that there is the involvement of signaling factors yet to be uncovered.

These many and complex signaling pathways act on transcription factors such as the forkhead (FOXO) and the Hsf transcription factors ***(148, 149)*** and nuclear receptors such as peroxisome proliferator-activated receptor alpha (PPAR$\alpha$) ***(150)*** so as to modulate the expression of genes. This modulation in gene expression acts to enhance protective and repair processes and to reduce the generation of harmful agents. It is proposed that through this complex series of events, CR extends life and slows the aging processes.

## References

1. McCay CM, Crowell MF, Maynard LA. The effect of retarded growth upon the length of life and upon the ultimate body size. J Nutr 1935;10:63–79.
2. Masoro, EJ. Caloric restriction: A key to understanding and modulating aging. Amsterdam: Elsevier, 2002.
3. Weindruch R, Walford RL. The retardation of aging and disease by dietary restriction. Springfield, IL: Charles C. Thomas, 1998.
4. Holehan AM, Merry BJ. The experimental manipulation of ageing by diet. Biol Rev 1986;61:329–69.
5. Pletcher SD, Khazaeli AA, Curtsinger JA. Why do life spans differ? Partitioning mean longevity differences in terms of age-specific mortality parameters. J Gerontol 2000;55A:B381–9.
6. Pugh TD, Oberly TD, Weindruch R. Dietary intervention at middle age: caloric restriction but not dehydroepiandrosterone sulfate increases lifespan and lifetime cancer incidence in mice. Cancer Res 1999;59:1642–8.
7. Finch CE. Longevity, senescence, and the genome. Chicago, IL: University of Chicago Press, 1990.
8. Driver C. A further comment on why the Gompertz plot does not measure aging. Biogerontology 2003;4:325–7.
9. Dhahbi JM, Kim HJ, Mote PL, Beaver RJ, Spindler SR. Temporal linkage between phenotype and genomic responses to caloric restriction. Proc Natl Acad Sci U S A 2004;101:5524–9.
10. Lipman RD, Smith DE, Blumberg J, Bronson RT. Effects of caloric restriction or augmentation in adult rats: Longevity and lesion biomarkers. Aging Clin Exp Res 1998;10:463–70.

11. Masoro EJ. Dietary restriction: An experimental approach to the study of the biology of aging. In: Masoro EJ, Austad SN, eds. Handbook of the biology of aging, 5th ed. San Diego, CA: Academic, 2001, pp. 396–420.
12. Liepa GU, Masoro EJ, Bertrand HA, Yu BP. Food restriction as a modulator of age-related changes in serum lipids. Am J Physiol 1980;238:E253–7.
13. Ward WF. Food restriction enhancement of the proteolytic capacity of aging rat liver. J Gerontol 1988;43:B121–4.
14. McClearn GE. Markers of aging. In: Birren JE, ed. Encyclopedia of gerontology, 2nd ed., vol. 2. San Diego, CA: Elsevier, 2007, pp. 117–24.
15. Maeda H, Gleiser CA, Masoro EJ, Murata I, McMahan CA, Yu BP. Nutritional influences on aging of Fischer 344 rats: II. Pathology. J Gerontol 1985;40:671–88.
16. Bronson RT, Lipman RD. Reduction in the rate of occurrence of age-related lesions in dietary restricted laboratory mice. Growth Dev Aging 1991;55:169–84.
17. Weindruch R. Dietary restriction, tumors, and aging in rodents. J Gerontol 1989;44(special issue):67–71.
18. Shimokawa I, Higami Y, Hubbard GB, McMahan CA, Masoro EJ, Yu BP. Diet and the suitability of the male Fischer 344 rat as a model for aging research. J Gerontol 1993;48:B27–32.
19. Mattson MP, Duan W, Lee J, Guo Z. Suppression of brain aging and neurodegenerative disorders by dietary restriction and environmental enrichment: molecular mechanisms. Mech Ageing Dev 2001;122:757–78.
20. Fernandes G, Yunis EJ, Miranda M, Smith J, Good RA. Nutritional inhibition of genetically determined renal disease and autoimmunity with prolongation of life in kdkd mice. Proc Natl Acad Sci U S A 1978;75:2888–92.
21. Wolf NS, Li Y, Pendergras W, Schmeider C, Turturro A. Normal mouse and rat strains as models for age-related cataract and the effect of caloric restriction on its development. Exp Eye Res 2000;70:683–92.
22. Sheldon WG, Warbritton AR, Bucci TJ, Tutturro A. Glaucoma in food restricted and ad libitum-fed DBA/2NNIA mice. Lab Anim Sci 1995;45:508–18.
23. Sheldon WG, Bucci TJ, Tuturro A. Thoracic apohyseal osteoarthritis in feed-restricted and ad libitum-fed B6C3F1mice. In: Mohr U, Dungworth D, Capen C, Carlton W, Sundberg J, Ward J, eds. Pathobiology of the aging mouse, vol 1. Washington, DC: ILSI, 1996, pp. 445–53.
24. Masoro EJ. Are age-associated diseases an integral part of aging? In Masoro EJ, Austad SM, eds. Handbook of the biology of aging, 6th ed. San Diego, CA: Elsevier, 2006, pp. 43–62.
25. McCay CM, Maynard LA, Sperling G, Barenes LL. Retarded growth, lifespan, ultimate body size, and age change in the albino rat after feeding diets restricted in calories. J Nutr 1939;18:1–13.
26. Masoro EJ, Iwaski K, Gleiser CA, McMahan CA, Seo E, Yu BP. Dietary modulation of the progression of nephropathy in aging rats: an evaluation of the importance of protein. Am J Clin Nutr 1989;49:1217–27.
27. Iwasaki K, Gleiser CA, Masoro EJ, McMahan CA, Seo E, Yu BP. Influence of restricting individual dietary components on longevity and age-related disease of Fischer rats: the fat component and the mineral component. J Gerontol 1998;43:B13–21.
28. Yu BP, Masoro EJ, Murata I, Bertrand HA, Lynd FT. Life span study of SPF Fischer 344 rats fed ad libitum or restricted diets: longevity, growth, lean body mass, and disease. J Gerontol 1982;37:130–41.
29. Zimmerman JA, Malloy V, Krojjcik R, Orentreich N. Nutritional control of aging. Exp Gerontol 2003;38:47–52.
30. Miller RA, Buehner G, Chang Y, Harper JM, Sigler R, Smith-Wheelock M. Methionine deficient diet extends mouse lifespan, slows immune and lens aging, alters glucose, T4, IGF-1 and insulin levels, and increases hepatocyte MIF levels and stress resistance. Aging Cell 2005;4:119–25.
31. Weindruch R, Walford RL. Dietary restriction in mice beginning at 1 year of age: effects on lifespan and spontaneous cancer incidence. Science 1982;215:1415–8.
32. Yu BP, Masoro EJ, McMahan CA. Life span study of SPF Fischer 344 male rats: I. Physical, metabolic, and longevity characteristics. J Gerontol 1985;40:657–70.

33. Bonkowski MS, Rocha JS, Masternak MM, Al Regaiey KA, Bartke A. Targeted disruption of growth hormone receptor interferes with the beneficial actions of caloric restriction. Proc Natl Acad Sci U S A 2006;103:7901–5.
34. Sonntag WE, Lenham JE, Ingram RL. Effects of aging and dietary restriction on tissue protein synthesis: Relationship to plasma insulin-like growth factor-1. J Gerontol 1992;47:B159–62.
35. Miller RA, Harper JM, Galecki A, Burke DT. Big mice die young: early life body weight predicts longevity in genetically heterogeneous mice. Aging Cell 2002;1:22–9.
36. Berg BN, Simms HS. Nutrition and longevity in the rat. II. Longevity and onset of disease with different levels of intake. J Nutr 1960;71:255–63.
37. Peeters A, Barendregt JJ, Willekins F, Mackenbach JP, Mamun AAI, Bonneux L. Obesity in adulthood and its consequences for life expectancy: A life-table analysis. Ann Intern Med 2003;138:E24–33.
38. Westman S. Development of the obese-hyperglycaemic syndrome in mice. Diabetologia 1968;4:141–9.
39. Garthwaite TL, Martinson DR, Tseng LF, Hagen TC, Menahan LA. A longitudinal hormonal profile of the genetically obese mouse. Endocrinology 1980;107:671–6.
40. Bertrand HA, Lynd FT, Masoro EJ, Yu BP. Changes in adipose mass and cellularity through the adult life of rats fed ad libitum or a life-prolonging restricted diet. J Gerontology 1980;35:827–35.
41. Harrison DE, Archer JR, Astle CM. Effects of food restriction on aging: separation of food intake and adiposity. Proc Natl Acad Sci U S A 1984;81:1835–8.
42. Barzilai N, Gupta GG. Revisiting the role of fat mass in life extension induced by caloric restriction. J Gerontol 1999;54A:B89–96.
43. Blüher M, Kahn BB, Kahn CR. Extended longevity in mice lacking the insulin receptor in adipose tissue. Science 2003;299:572–4.
44. Blüher M, Michael MD, Peroni OD, et al. Adipose tissue selective insulin receptor knockout protects against obesity and obesity-related glucose intolerance. Dev Cell 2002;3:25–38.
45. Moitra J, Mason MM, Olive M, et al. Life without white fat: a transgenic mouse. Genes Dev 1998;12:3168–81.
46. Ross SR, Graves RA, Spiegelman BM. Targeted expression of a toxin gene to adipose tissue: transgenic mice resistant to obesity. Genes Dev 1993;7:1318–24.
47. Shimomura I, Hammer RE, Richardson JA, et al. Insulin resistance and diabetes mellitus in transgenic mice expressing nuclear SREBP-1c in adipose tissue: model for congenital generalized lipodystrophy. Genes Dev 1998;12:3182–94.
48. Benedict FG. Vital energetics. A study in comparative basal metabolism. Publication 503. Washington, DC: Carnegie Institute of Washington, 1938, pp. 1–215.
49. Garrow JS. Energy balance and obesity in man. Oxford: Elsevier/North Holland, 1978, p. 195.
50. Sacher GA. Life table modification and life prolongation. In: Finch C, Hayflick L, eds. Handbook of the biology of aging. New York: Van Nootrand Reinhold, 1977, pp. 582–638.
51. Pearl R. The rate of living. New York, NY: Alfred Knopf, 1928, p. 185.
52. Harman D. Ageing: a theory based on free radical and radiation chemistry. J Gerontol 1956;11:298–300.
53. Cutler R. Antioxidants, aging and longevity. In: Pryor WA, ed. Free radicals in biology, vol. 6. Orlando, FL: Academic Press, 1984, p. 381.
54. Blanc S, Schoeller D, Kemnitz J, et al. Energy expenditure of rhesus monkeys subjected to 11 years of dietary restriction. J Clin Endocrinol Metab 2003;88:16–23.
55. Dulloo AG, Giradier L. 24 Hour energy expenditure several months after weight loss in the underfed rat: evidence for a chronic increase in whole-body metabolic efficiency. Int J Obes Relat Metab Disord 1993;17:115–23.
56. Lane MA, Baer DJ, Rumpler WV, et al. Calorie restriction lowers body temperature in rhesus monkey, consistent with a postulated anti-aging mechanism in rodents. Proc Natl Acad Sci U S A 1996;93:4159–64.
57. Beckman KB, Ames BN. The free radical theory of aging matures. Physiol Rev 1998;78:547–81.

58. Barja G. Rate of generation of oxidative stress-related damage and animal longevity. Free Radic Biol Med 2002;33:1167–72.
59. Bevilacqua L, Ramsey JJ, Hagopian K, Weindruch R, Harper ME. Long-term caloric restriction increases UCP3 content but decreases proton leak and reactive oxygen species production in rat skeletal muscle mitochondria. Am J Physiol Endocrinol Metab 2005;280:E429–38.
60. McCarter R, Shimokawa A, Ikeno Y, et al. Physical activity as a factor in the action of dietary restriction on aging: Effects in Fischer 344 rats. Aging (Milano) 1997;9:73–9.
61. Masoro EJ, Yu BP, Bertrand H. Action of food restriction in delaying the aging processes. Proc Natl Acad Sci U S A 1982;79:4239–41.
62. McCarter RJ, Palmer J. Energy metabolism and aging: a lifelong study in Fischer 344 rats. Am J Physiol 1992;263:E448–52.
63. Speakman JR, Talbot DA, Selman C, et al. Uncoupled and surviving: individual mice with high metabolism have greater mitochondrial uncoupling and live longer. Aging Cell 2004;3:87–95.
64. Selman C, Phillips T, Staib JL, Duncan JS, Leeuwenburgh C, Speakman JR. Energy expenditure of calorically restricted rats is higher than predicted from their altered body composition. Mech Ageing Dev 2005;126:783–93.
65. Lambert AJ, Merry BJ. Lack of effect of caloric restriction on bioenergetics and reactive oxygen species production in intact rat hepatocytes. J Gerontol A Biol Sci Med Sci 2005;60A:175–80.
66. McCarter RJ, Masoro EJ, Yu BP. Rat muscle structure and metabolism in relation to age and food intake. Am J Physiol 1982;242:R89–93.
67. Gonzalez-Pacheco DM, Buss WC, Koehler KM, Woodside WF, Alpert SS. Energy restriction reduces metabolic rate in adult male Fisher-344 rats. J Nutr 1993;123:90–7.
68. Austad SN, Fischer KE. Mammalian aging, metabolism and ecology: evidence from the bats and marsupials. J Gerontol 1991;46:B47–53.
69. Gerschman R, Gilbert DL, Nye SW, Dwyer P, Fenn WO. Oxygen poisoning and X-irrradiation: a mechanism in common. Science 1954;119:623–26.
70. Commoner B, Townsend J, Pake GE. Free radicals in biological materials. Nature 1954;174:689–91.
71. Wallace DC. Mitochondrial defects in neurodegenerative disease. Ment Retard Dev Disabil Res Rev 2001;7:158–66.
72. Austad SN. Vertebrate aging research. Aging Cell 2007;6:135–8.
73. VanRemmen H, Ikeno Y, Hamilton M, et al. Life-long reduction in MnSOD activity results in increased DNA damage and higher incidence of cancer but does not accelerate aging. Physiol Genomics 2003;16:29–37.
74. Huang TT, Carlson EJ, Gillespie AM, Shi Y, Epstein CJ. 2000. Ubiquitous overexpression of CuZn superoxide dismutase does not extend life span in mice. J Gerontol A Biol Sci Med Sci 2000;55:85–9.
75. Schriner SE, Linford NJ, Martin GM, et al. Extension of murine life span by overexpression of catalase targeted to mitochondria. Science 2005;308:1909–11.
76. Andziak B, O'Connor TP, Qi W, et al. High oxidative damage levels in the longest-living rodent, the naked mole-rat. Aging Cell 2006;5:463–71.
77. Shigenaga MK, Hagen TM, Ames BN. Oxidative damage and mitochondrial decay in aging. Proc Natl Acad Sci U S A 1994;91:10771–8.
78. De AK, Chipalkatti S, Aiyar AS. Some biochemical parameters of ageing in relation to dietary protein. Mech Ageing Dev 1983;21:37–48.
79. Chipalkatti S, De AK, Aiyar AS. Effect of diet restriction on some biochemical parameters related to aging in mice. J Nutr 1983;113:944–50.
80. Laganiere S, Yu BP. Effect of chronic food restriction in aging rats I. Liver subcellular membranes. Mech Ageing Dev 1989;48:207–19.
81. Laganiere S, Yu BP. Anti-lipoperoxidation action of food restriction. Biochem Biophys Res Commun 1987;145:1185–91.
82. Merry BJ. Calorie restriction and age-related stress. In: Toussaint O, Osiewacz HD, Lithgow G, Brack C, eds. Molecular and cellular gerontology. New York, NY: New York Academy of Sciences, 2002, pp. 180–98.

83. Dubey A, Forster M, Harbans L, Sohal RS. Effect of age and caloric intake on protein oxidation in different brain regions and on behavioral functions of the mouse. Arch Biochem Biophys 1996;333:189–97.
84. Lass A, Sohal BH, Weindruch R, Forster MJ, Sohal RS. Caloric restriction prevents age-associated accrual of oxidative damage to mouse skeletal muscle mitochondria. Free Radic Biol Med 1998;25:1089–97.
85. Kaneko T, Tahara S, Matsuo M. Retarding effect of dietary restriction on the accumulation of 8-hydroxy-2'-deoxyguanosine in organs of Fischer 344 rats during aging. Free Radic Biol Med 1997;23:76–81.
86. Kang CM, Krystal BS, Yu BP. Age-related mitochondrial DNA deletions: effect of dietary restriction. Free Radic Biol Med 1998;24:148–54.
87. Muller FJ, Lustgarten MS, Jang Y, Richardson A, VanRemmen H. Trends in oxidative aging theories. Free Radic Biol Med 2007;43:477–503.
88. Merry BJ. Oxidative stress and mitochondrial function with aging – the effects of calorie restriction. Aging Cell 2004;3:7–12.
89. Cerami A. Hypothesis: glucose as a mediator of aging. J Am Geriatr Soc 1985;33:626–34.
90. Kassi E, Papavassiliou AG. Could glucose be a proaging factor? J Cell Mol Med 2008;12:1194–8.
91. Masoro EJ, Katz MS, McMahan CA. Evidence for the glycation hypothesis of aging from the food restricted rodent model. J Gerontol 1989;44:B20–2.
92. Monnier VM. Nonenzymatic glycosylation, the Maillard Reaction and the aging process. J Gerontol 1990;45:B105–11.
93. Sell DR, Monnier VM. Long-lived proteins: extracellular matrix and lens crystallins. In: Masoro EJ, ed. Handbook of physiology: section II, aging. New York, NY: Oxford University Press, 1995, pp. 235–308.
94. Cai W, He JC, Zhu L, Chen X, Striker GE, Vlassara H. AGE-receptor-1 counteracts cellular oxidant stress induced by AGEs via negative regulation of p66shc-dependent FKHRL1 phosphorylation. Am J Physiol Cell Physiol 2008;294:C145–52.
95. Yan SF, D'Agati V, Schmidt AM, Ramasamy R. Receptor for advanced glycation endproducts (RAGE): a formidable force in the pathogenesis of the cardiovascular complications of diabetes and aging. Curr Mol Med 2007;7:699–710.
96. McCarter RJ, Mejia W, Ikeno Y, et al. Plasma glucose and the action of calorie restriction on aging. J Gerontol A Biol Sci Med Sci 2007;62A:1059–70.
97. Masoro EJ, McCarter RJ, Katz MS, McMahan CA. Dietary restriction alters characteristics of glucose fuel use. J Gerontol 1992;47:B202–8.
98. Bergman RN. Toward physiological understanding of glucose tolerance. Minimal model approach. Diabetes 1989;38:1512–27.
99. Kenyon C, Chang J, Gensch A, Rudner A, Tabtiang R. A C. elegans mutant that lives twice as long as the wild type. Nature 1993;366:461–4.
100. Clancy DJ, Gems D, Harshman LG, et al. Extension of life span by loss of CHICO, a Drosophila insulin receptor substrate protein. Science 2001;292:104–6.
101. Tatar M, Kopelman A, Epstein D, et al. A mutant Drosophila insulin receptor homolog that extends life span and impairs neuroendocrine function. Science 2001;292:107–10.
102. Gupta G, Li S, Ma X-H, et al. Aging does not contribute to the decline in insulin action on storage of muscle glycogen in rats. Am J Physiol 2000;278:111–7.
103. Iida KT, Shimano H, Kawakami Y, et al. Insulin up-regulates tumor necrosis factor-alpha in macrophages through extracellular-regulated kinase-dependent pathway. J Biol Chem 2001;276:32531–7.
104. Biddinger SB, Kahn CR. From mice to men: insights into the insulin resistance syndromes. Annu Rev Physiol 2000;68:123–58.
105. Taguchi A, Wartschow LM, White MF. Brain IRS2 signaling coordinates life span and nutrient homeostasis. Science 2007;317:369–72.
106. Dean DJ, Brozinick JT Jr, Cushman SW, Cartee GD. Calorie restriction increases cell surface GLUT-4 in insulin-stimulated skeletal muscle. Am J Physiol 1998;275:E957–64.

107. Swanson DR. Somatomedin C and arginine: implicit connections between mutually isolated literatures. Perspect Biol Med 1990;33:157–86.
108. Kelijman M. Age-related alterations of the growth hormone/insulin-like-growth-factor I axis. J Am Geriatr Soc 1991;39:295–307.
109. Laron Z, Doron M, Arnikan B. Plasma growth hormone in men and women over 70 years of age. Med Sport Phys Activity Aging 1970;4:126–9.
110. Corpas E, Harman SM, Blackman MR. Human growth hormone and human aging. Endocr Rev 1993;14:20–39.
111. Sonntag WE, Steger RW, Forman LJ, Meites J. Decreased pulsatile release of growth hormone in old male rats. Endocrinology 1980;107:1875–9.
112. Florini JR, Harned JA, Richman RA, Weiss JP. Effect of rat age on serum levels of growth hormone and somatomedins. Mech Ageing Dev 1981;15:165–76.
113. Holzenberger M, Dupont J, Ducos B, et al. IGF-1 receptor regulates lifespan and resistance to oxidative stress in mice. Nature 2003;21:182–7.
114. Coschigano KT, Clemmons D, Bellush LL, Kopchick JJ. Assessment of growth parameters and lifespan of GHR/BP gene-disrupted mice. Endocrinology 2000;141:2608–13.
115. Flurkey K, Papaconstantinou J, Miller RA, Harrison DE. Lifespan extension and delayed immune and collagen aging in mutant mice with defects in growth hormone production. Proc Natl Acad Sci U S A 2001;98:6736–41.
116. Brown-Borg HM, Borg KE, Meliska CJ, Bartke A. Dwarf mice and the aging process. Nature 1996;384:33.
117. Hursting SD, Switzer BR, French JE, Kari FW. The growth hormone: insulin-like growth factor-1 axis is a mediator of diet restriction-induced inhibition of mononuclear cell leukemia in Fischer rats. Cancer Res 1993;53:2750–7.
118. Breese CR, Ingram RL, Sonntag WE. Influence of age and long-term dietary restriction on plasma insulin-like growth factor-1 (IGF-1), IGF-1 gene expression, and IGF-1 binding proteins. J Gerontol 1991;46:B180–7.
119. D'Costa AP, Lenham JE, Ingram RL, Sonntag WE. Moderate caloric restriction increases type 1 IGF-1 receptors and protein synthesis in aging rats. Mech Aging Dev 1993;71:59–71.
120. Sonntag WE, Lynch CD, Cefalu WT, et al. Pleiotropic effects of growth hormone and insulin-like growth factor (IGF-1) on biological aging: inferences from moderate caloric-restricted animals. J Gerontol 1999;54A:B521–38.
121. Masoro EJ. Hormesis and the antiaging action of dietary restriction. Exp Gerontol 1998;33:61–6.
122. Turturro A, Hass B, Hart RW. Hormesis: implications for risk assessment caloric intake (body weight) as an exemplar. Hum Exp Toxicol 1998;17:454–9.
123. Calebrese EJ, Baldwin LA. Hormesis as a biological hypothesis. Environ Health Perspect 1998;106(suppl 1):357–62.
124. Caratero A, Courtade M, Bonnet L, Planel H, Caratero C. Effect of continuous gamma irradiation at very low dose on the life span of mice. Gerontology 1998;44:272–6.
125. Mattson MP. Hormesis defined. Ageing Res Rev 2008;7:1–7.
126. Rattan SIS. Applying hormesis in aging research and therapy. Hum Exp Toxicol 2001;20:281–5.
127. Munck CV, Guyre PM, Holbrook NJ. Physiologic functions of glucocorticoids in stress and their relation to pharmacological actions. Endocr Rev 1984;5:25–44.
128. Sabatino F, Masoro EJ, McMahan CA, Kuhn RW. An assessment of the role of the glucocorticoid system in aging processes and in the action of food restriction. J Gerontol 1991;46:B171–9.
129. Klebanov S, Shehab D, Stavinoha WB, Yongman S, Nelson JF. Hyperadrenocorticism attenuated inflammation and the life-prolonging action of food restriction in mice. J Gerontol 1995;50A:B78–82.
130. Heydari AR, Wu B, Takahashi R, Strong R, Richardson A. Expression of heat shock protein 70 is altered by age and diet at the level of transcription. Mol Cell Biol 1993;13:2900–18.
131. Duffy PH, Feuers FJ, Pipkin JL, et al. The effect of dietary restriction and aging on physiological response to drugs. In: Hart RW, Neuman DA, Robertson RT, eds. Dietary restriction:

implications for the design and interpretation of toxicity and carcinogenicity studies. Washington, DC: ILSI, 1995, pp. 125–40.
132. Keenan KP, Ballam GC, Dixit R, et al. The effect of diet, overfeeding and moderate dietary restriction on Sprague–Dawley rat survival, disease, and toxicology. J Nutr 1997;127(suppl):851S–6S.
133. Rattan SIS. Aging, anti-aging, and hormesis. Mech Ageing Dev 2004;125:285–9.
134. Crypser JR, Johnson TE. Multiple stressors in Caenorhabditis elegans induced stress hormesis and extended longevity. J Gerontol 2002;57:B109–14.
135. Martin GM, Austad SN, Johnson TE. Genetic analysis of ageing: role of oxidative damage and environmental stresses. Nat Genet 1996;13:25–34.
136. Oster MH, Fiedler PJ, Levin N, Cronin MJ. Adaptation of growth hormone and insulin-like growth factor-1 axis to chronic and severe calorie or protein malnutrition. J Clin Invest 1995;95:2258–65.
137. Dillmann WH, Berry S, Alexander N, A physiological dose of triiodothyronine normalizes cardiac myosin adenosine triphosphatase activity and changes myosin isoenzyme distribution in semistarved rats. Endocrinology 1983;112:2081–7.
138. Sabatino F, Masoro EJ, McMahan CA, Kuhn RW. An assessment of the role of the glucocorticoid system in aging processes and in the action of food restriction. J Gerontol 1991;46:B171–9.
139. Tomita M, Shimokawa I, Higami Y, et al. Modulation by dietary restriction in gene expression related to insulin-like growth factor-1 in rat muscle. Aging Clin Exp Res 2001;13:273–81.
140. Herlihy JT, Stacy C, Bertrand HA. Long-term food restriction depresses serum thyroid concentration in the rat. Mech Ageing Dev 1990;53:9–16.
141. Richardson A, McCarter RJM. Mechanism of food restriction: Change of rate or change of set point. In: Ingram DK, Baker GT III, Shock NW, eds. Nutritional modulation of aging processes. Trumbull, CT: Food and Nutrition Press, 1991, pp. 193–204.
142. Sinclair DA, Horwitz KT. Dietary restriction, hormesis, and small molecule mimetics. In: Masoro EJ, Austad DN, eds. Handbook of the biology of aging, 6th ed. San Diego, CA: Elsevier, 2006, pp. 63–104.
143. Kennedy BK, Steffen KK, Kaeberlein M. Ruminations on dietary restriction and aging. Cell Mol Life Sci 2007;64:1323–8.
144. Cohen HY, Miller C, Bitterman KJ, et al. Calorie restriction promotes mammalian cell survival by inducing the SIRT1 deacetylase. Science 2004;305:390–2.
145. Corton JF, Brown-Borg HM. Peroxisome proliferator-activated receptor gamma coactivator 1 in caloric restriction. J Gerontol 2005;60A:1494–509.
146. Nemoto S, Fergusson MM, Finkel T. Nutrient availability regulates SIRT1 through a forkhead-dependent pathway. Science 2004;306:2105–8.
147. Mori K, Yahata K, Mukoyama M, et al. Disruption of klotho gene causes an abnormal energy homeostasis response in mice. Biochem Biophys Res Commun 2000;278:665–70.
148. Wang F, Nguyen M, Qin FX, Tong Q. SIRT2 deacetylates FOXO3a in response to oxidative stress and caloric restriction. Aging Cell 2007;6:505–14.
149. Cohen E, Bieschke J, Perciavalle RM, Kelly JW, Dillin A. Opposing activities protect against age-onset proteotoxicity. Science 2006;313:1604–10.
150. Corton JC, Apte U, Anderson SP, et al. Mimetics of caloric restriction include agonists of lipid-activated nuclear receptors. J Biol Chem 2004;279:46204–12.

# Chapter 7
# Growth Hormone and Aging in Mice

**Holly M. Brown-Borg, Sunita Sharma, Kurt E. Borg, and Sharlene G. Rakoczy**

**Abstract** After decades of research, the physiological mechanisms leading to aging are still poorly understood. A number of studies have shown that the endocrine system is intimately involved in the control of aging processes. The somatotropic axis, in particular, has come to the forefront as a major player in aging and longevity. Many of these reports derive data from multiple endocrine mutants, those that exhibit elevated levels of both growth hormone (GH) and insulin-like growth factor I (IGF-I) or deficiencies in one or both of these hormones. In general, both spontaneous and genetically engineered GH and IGF-I deficiencies have led to small body size, delayed development of both sexual maturation and age-related pathologic conditions, and life-span extension. In contrast, high levels of circulating GH have led to larger body sizes, early puberty and reproductive senescence, increased cancer incidence, and reduced life span compared with wild-type animals with normal plasma hormone concentrations. This information, along with that found in multiple other species, implicates this anabolic pathway as the major regulator of longevity in animals.

**Keywords** Insulin-like growth factor I • longevity • metabolism • stress resistance • reproduction

**Abbreviations** CR: Caloric restriction; GH: Growth hormone: GHa; Growth hormone antagonist; GHRKO: growth hormone receptor/binding protein knockout; GHRH: Growth hormone releasing hormone; GPX: Glutathione peroxidase; GSH: Glutathione; IGF-I: Insulin-like growth factor I; IGF-IR: insulin-like growth factor I receptor; IR: Insulin receptor; LD50: Lethal dose, 50%; LID: Liver-specific IGF-I deletion; PRL: Prolactin; ROS: Reactive oxygen species; SOD: Superoxide dismutase; TSH: Thyrotropin

---

H.M. Brown-Borg (✉), S. Sharma, K.E. Borg, and S.G. Rakoczy
University of North Dakota, School of Medicine and Health Sciences, Grand Forks, ND, USA
e-mail: brownbrg@medicine.nodak.edu

C. Sell et al. (eds.), *Life-Span Extension*, Aging Medicine,
DOI 10.1007/978-1-60327-507-1_7,

## 7.1 Introduction

The factors that regulate aging processes and life span are poorly understood. However, hormones of the pituitary gland continue to receive the overall attention of researchers in the field and have a long-standing history of being key players in aging and longevity. Nearly 70 years have passed since Mulinos and Pomerantz *(1)* published a paper indicating that food restriction inhibited the secretion of several pituitary hormones in rats. Decades later, Everitt and coworkers *(2)* showed that hypophysectomy resulted in improvements in age-related pathologic changes of rats. These investigators confirmed and extended previous work and showed that food restriction reduced pituitary hormone release, delayed onset of age-related disease, and extended life span *(3)*. It was then postulated that the pituitary gland produced antiaging factors. Continued work by Everitt and colleagues *(4)* showed that, in rats, both hypophysectomy and caloric restriction (CR) similarly retarded tail tendon collagen aging, abolished age-related proteinuria, and delayed the onset of several age-related conditions such as total tumor incidence, hind limb paralysis, aortic wall thickening, and cardiac and kidney enlargement. On the basis of these studies, it was believed that pituitary hormones played a significant role in life span regulation. In agreement with these ideas, an extension of life span was recently shown following hypophysectomy in adult mice *(5)*.

The anterior pituitary produces and secretes multiple hormones, but the most well studied of these hormones with regard to aging and longevity is growth hormone (GH) and its downstream effector, insulin-like growth factor I (IGF-I). The somatotropic axis in mammals as it relates to aging processes and life span is considered in this chapter. The somatotropic axis consists of hypothalamic hormones, growth hormone, the IGFs, and downstream signaling molecules. It is the balance between the two hypothalamic factors, growth hormone releasing hormone (GHRH) and somatostatin, that determines the rate of GH production and secretion from the anterior pituitary.

Plasma GH directly stimulates IGF-I production and secretion by the liver in addition to exerting direct effects on other tissues. Local tissue production of GH or IGF-I also occurs, suggesting the importance of the autocrine and paracrine actions of these hormones. Growth hormone and IGF-I have both somatic effects that stimulate the growth of tissues and metabolic effects that play a role in protein, carbohydrate, and lipid metabolism. Alterations in these interrelated pathways can thus lead to growth retardation or tissue proliferation and a variety of metabolic disturbances. It is well documented that GH levels begin to decline soon after the peripubertal period of rapid growth *(6)*. The progressive decline of GH secretion with age has been termed the somatopause in humans and has also been shown to occur in rodents *(7)*. Plasma IGF-I levels decrease in parallel with the decline in GH pulses *(8)*. The lower levels of plasma GH and IGF-I in elderly humans are thought to cause many aspects of physical change in aging including decreased muscle mass, strength, skin thickness, and bone mineral density and increased fat mass and overall loss of energy. In rodents, a significant body of literature has been generated showing that GH and IGF-I affect multiple physiological systems leading to alterations in age-related pathologic changes and life span. Both spontaneous and genetically engineered GH and IGF-I mutant mice have been studied. The physiological factors affected by deficiencies or excesses of GH or related molecules are significant and include body size, metabolism, reproduction, and stress resistance and contribute to an overall effect on life span.

## 7.2 Life Span

Several types of GH/IGF mutant mice have been studied: the Ames dwarf, Snell dwarf, GH receptor/binding protein knockout (*GHRKO*), Little, Midi, GH receptor antagonist, IGF receptor knockdown, liver specific *Igf*-1 deletion (LID), and GH transgenic mice (Table 7.1). Each of these mutants is described in the context of life span followed by specific information regarding possible mechanisms of delayed and premature aging.

Ames dwarf mice live 49% (males) to 68% (females) longer than wild-type control mice (average life span, 24 months) ***(9)***. Ames mice have a primary pituitary deficiency resulting in the absence of GH, prolactin (PRL), and thyrotropin (TSH). These deficiencies result from a point mutation in the *prop-1* gene that promotes appropriate differentiation of the pituitary cells into somatotrophs, lactotrophs, and thyrotrophs ***(10, 11)***. As a consequence of the GH deficiency, these mice have undetectable levels of plasma IGF-I ***(12)***. Ames mice exhibit delayed aging and are one of the longest living endocrine mutants. In addition, CR produces a further extension of life span of Ames mice ***(13)***.

Snell dwarf mice are phenotypically identical to Ames mice; they lack GH, PRL, and TSH ***(14)*** owing to lack of normal pituitary differentiation because of a mutation in the transcription factor *pit-1* (downstream of *prop-1*) ***(15)***. These mice also live longer (40–45%) than normal littermates and have significantly reduced plasma IGF-I levels ***(16)***. Studies examining hormone replacement in Snell dwarf mice demonstrated that short-term (11 weeks) GH and thyroxine replacement did not affect longevity. However, thyroxine administration throughout adult life did shorten life span significantly ***(17)***. Replacing PRL in dwarf mice shortened life span in one study but had no affect on longevity in another (Bartke, unpublished observations) ***(16)***. Therefore, the lack of GH and IGF-I are proposed as the main mediators of the life span extension in these mice.

More evidence that reduced levels of GH/IGF-I lead to life extension is derived from GH receptor/binding protein knockout mice (GHRKO) ***(18)***. These mice have high levels of plasma GH but significantly reduced levels of IGF-I because of the lack of receptor binding in target tissues. The GHRKO mice exhibit delayed puberty and an average increase in life span of 31–46% ***(19, 20)*** compared with wild-type animals. Little mice possess a spontaneous mutation in the GHRH receptor ***(21–23)***. These mice are deficient in GH, but only a 25% increase in life span is observed when they are fed a low-fat diet compared with wild-type controls ***(16)***.

**Table 7.1** Phenotypic characteristics of GH/IGF-1 long-living mutant rodent

| Phenotype | Ames (prop-1) | Snell (pit-1) | GHR KO | Igf-IR +/- | LID | Little (GHRHR mutant) | Klotho | Midi (IGF-I hypomorph) |
|---|---|---|---|---|---|---|---|---|
| GH/Igf-I/ Insulin signaling | ↓ | ↓ | ↓ | ↓ | ↓ | ↓ | ↓ | ↓ |
| Body size | ↓ | ↓ | ↓ | ↓ | ↔ | ↓ | ↔ | ↓ |
| Reproduction | ↓ | ↓ | ↓ | ↔ | ↔ | ↓ | ↓ | |
| Insulin sensitivity | ↑ | ↑ | ↑ | Partially IGF-I resistant | Insulin resistant | NK | Insulin and IGF-I resistant | NK |
| Stress resistance | ↑ | ↑ | ↑ | ↑ | NK | NK | ↑ | NK |
| Longevity | 35%-70% ↑ | 42% ↑ | 42%-55% ↑ | 33% females ↑ | ↔ | 25% ↑ | 18%-30% ↑ | ↑ |

*GH* growth hormone, *IGF-I* insulin-like growth factor-I, *LID* liver IGF-I mutant, *NK* not known

Mice engineered to express a GH antagonist (mutated bovine GH) phenotypically resemble Little mice but do not live longer than their normal counterparts, even though they have greatly reduced levels of IGF-I ***(20, 24)***.

IGF mutants have been more difficult to engineer with several early attempts resulting in embryonic lethality. A 42% postnatal survival rate in mice created to lack *Igf-1* gene expression was reported with severely retarded growth both in utero and postnatally (35% at birth and 65% as adults) ***(25–27)***. No life-span data have been reported in these mice. However, mice with a 50% reduction in IGF-I receptor expression (*Igf-1* receptor knockdown) lived 26% longer than normal mice, although the reported life span of the normal mice was relatively short (19 months) ***(28)***. Liver-specific *Igf-1* gene deletion (LID) mice have a 75% reduction in circulating IGF-I levels yet do not live longer than wild-type control mice ***(29, 30)***. Midi mice, which express a hypomorphic *Igf-1* allele, exhibit 50–60% reductions in circulating IGF-I levels and have recently been reported to live longer than wild-type mice (Sell, personal communication). Mice with impaired IGF-I signaling (Klotho mice) live 19–25% longer than normal mice ***(31)***. The evidence is overwhelming and clearly demonstrates that reduced GH/IGF-I signaling via reductions in plasma GH/IGF-I hormone levels or altered hormone receptor interactions extends life span in rodents.

## 7.3 Mechanisms Contributing to Aging Processes

### *7.3.1 Growth and Body Size*

Somatic growth is driven by GH and IGF-I; thus body and organ size differences are observed in many of the endocrine mutants. Many mice and rats with reduced signaling of these pathways are significantly smaller than wild-type animals, a phenotype closely associated with longevity. IGF-I receptor knockdown mice are slightly smaller (8% in males) than wild-type mice, whereas Ames and Snell dwarf mice are 66% smaller (both sexes; one third the size of wild-type mice) ***(14, 28)***. Growth hormone receptor knockout mice are 40% the size of wild-type siblings as adults ***(19)*** and Little mice featuring a mutated GHRH receptor gene are 33% smaller than normal mice in body size. Midi mice express a hypomorphic IGF-I allele and exhibit a reduction in body weight in comparison with wild-type mice, a function of the 50% reduction in plasma IGF-I concentrations (Sell, personal communication). Two strains of dwarf rats also exhibit growth deficiencies. Antisense GH transgenic rats are 25% smaller and dw/dw rats at 3 months of age are 40% smaller than their wild-type counterparts ***(32–34)***. LID mice do not differ in size from wild-type mice and exhibit normal parameters of growth and development with only one quarter of wild-type circulating IGF-I levels ***(29)***. However, when LID mice are crossed with mice overexpressing a GH antagonist (GHa) to inactivate GH, the LID x GHa mice are 44% smaller than the LID mice and 30% smaller than control mice ***(35)***. Data exist showing that body size in other mammals, dogs in particular, but also in horses and likely in humans, plays a role in the determination of life span ***(36–38)***. The relationship between small body size and longevity is further supported by reports showing that mice selected for reduced body sizes live longer ***(39)***; it is also known that CR reduces growth and adult body size ***(40)***.

In contrast to animals with GH or IGF-I deficiencies, animals overexpressing GH are significantly larger (30–60%) and exhibit shorter life spans than wild-type controls ***(41–43)***. In a recent analysis, de Magalhaes and colleagues ***(44)*** showed that GH and the GH receptor statistically influenced aging whereas IGF-I receptor (IGF-IR) and the insulin receptor did not. Therefore, growth negatively influences life span in mammals, suggesting that GH is the most important mediator of postnatal growth ***(45)***.

### 7.3.2 Reproduction

Growth hormone and IGF-I are known to affect development of numerous organ systems; therefore, lifelong deficiencies or excesses produce secondary endocrine alterations. Specifically, reproductive organ development and function are impaired when serum GH or IGF-I concentrations are abnormal (***46***, extensive review). IGF-I deficiency, as exhibited by GHRKO mice, results in delayed sexual maturation but most animals are fertile. Normal fertility is also observed in LID, Midi, and IGF-IR heterozygote mice, each of which have significant reductions in IGF-I levels or in the ability to respond to this hormone ***(28, 29)***. Furthermore, mice lacking IGF-I altogether, as in IGF-I null mice, are sterile ***(46, 47)***. On the surface, corresponding data in Ames and Snell dwarf mice also suggest that a total lack of peripheral IGF-I results in sterility. However, ectopic pituitary placement (donor pituitary in renal capsule secreting PRL) restores fertility in females whereas short-term thyroxine replacement enhances already subfertile dwarf male reproductive behavior and success. Gonadal dysfunction in these animals is dependent on background strain ***(48)***. Of course, both Snell and Ames mice had additional underlying endocrine dysfunction, lacking both circulating PRL and TSH. Female Little mice, also deficient in GH, exhibit delayed sexual maturation whereas males are considered subfertile because of defects in sexual behavior ***(49)***. In dw/dw rats lacking IGF-I, fertility is also considered subnormal, with the males exhibiting small testes and impaired sperm motility ***(50, 51)***. IGF-I resistance also results in reduced fertility ***(31)***. Concomitant with lower plasma IGF-I levels, calorie-restricted rodents display delayed puberty, reduction in litter size, and lower fecundity ***(52–54)***. Evaluation of GH deficiency without altered IGF-I has not been possible to date. However, when plasma GH levels are significantly elevated, both sexual maturation and reproductive senescence occur earlier, as found in GH transgenic mice ***(55–57)***. Excess bovine GH seems to have little effect on male fertility, although senescence does occur earlier ***(56)***. The degree of suppression appears to be dependent on the levels of plasma GH ***(42, 56, 58)***. Chandrashekar and coworkers ***(59)*** suggest that many of the GH effects on the reproductive system are due to alterations in IGF-I concentrations and actions leading to the reproductive anomalies described in GH/IGF-I mutants.

### 7.3.3 Metabolism

Hormonal regulation of metabolic pathways is a key determinant of longevity. The actions of GH on glucose regulation are well known. This hormone is a diabetogenic factor in that it opposes the actions of insulin. GH elevates plasma glucose concentrations by stimulating gluconeogenesis and glycogenolysis and inhibiting glucose uptake at the tissue level. Therefore, elevated GH levels such as those observed in acromegalic patients and genetically engineered mice with elevated plasma GH levels exhibit hyperinsulinemia, hyperglycemia, and/or insulin resistance ***(60, 61)***. More than 50% of humans with supraphysiological GH levels become diabetic and develop microvascular and macrovascular complications associated with hyperglycemia. In sharp contrast, reduced insulin secretion and enhanced insulin sensitivity are hallmarks of longevity in mutant mice ***(61–64)***. Insulin sensitivity declines with age and is related to visceral fat stores in that sensitivity increases when visceral fat decreases ***(65, 66)***. The plasma of GH-deficient (Ames and Snell) and GH-resistant (GHRKO dwarf) mice is low in both glucose and insulin, and the animals are very insulin sensitive ***(62–64, 67)***. The enhanced insulin sensitivity in dwarf mice results in part from elevated levels of insulin receptors (GHRKO mice) and elevations in IRS-1 and IRS-2 (downstream effectors of IR) in Ames mice ***(62, 68)***. In addition, glucose utilization, gluconeogenesis, and glycogenolysis are significantly decreased in Snell dwarf mice ***(69)***. Furthermore, Ames mice have lower numbers of pancreatic islet cells ***(70)***.

Low levels of IGF-I can also lead to insulin resistance, as found in both male IGF-IR heterozygous mice and in liver IGF-I deletion mice ***(28, 30, 71)***. The insulin resistance results from GH hypersecretion because the actions of GH are inactivated in the LID x GHa animals and these animals are insulin sensitive ***(35)***. Taken together, the bulk of the data suggests that IGF-I plays a smaller role metabolically, likely fine tuning GH and insulin activities, some of which may occur via IGF-I binding to insulin receptors and direct effects on adipose tissue. Mechanistically reducing circulating glucose throughout life probably delays aging by decreasing the accumulation of detrimental processes associated with glycation end products, slowing metabolism, and reducing the associated reactive oxygen species (ROS) generation ***(72, 73)***.

Insulin sensitivity declines with age ***(74)***. FIRKO mice, which lack the insulin receptor in fat tissue, exhibit significantly reduced fat mass and increased insulin sensitivity and are protected against age-related obesity. The decrease in fat mass occurs in the absence of reduced food intake. These mice do not develop diabetes or glucose intolerance and, importantly, live 18% longer than wild-type control mice ***(75, 76)***. Although studies of centenarians have not yet shown statistical differences in IGF-I levels, greatly enhanced insulin sensitivity is strongly correlated with longevity in this unique population ***(77, 78)***. The effects of GH and IGF-I on metabolism are apparent in mutant rodents and humans and provide additional clues as to the role of these hormones in aging and longevity.

### *7.3.4 Stress Resistance*

The somatotropic axis also affects an organism's overall resistance to stress. Stress resistance in GH/IGF-I mutant mice was covered extensively in a recent review ***(79)***; therefore, just an overview is included in this report. The components of this system are more diffuse and include the heat shock proteins, cellular repair factors, phase II detoxification proteins, antioxidants, metal chelators, and factors that prevent or suppress tumor growth. Resistance to oxidative stress, which is significantly affected by altered signaling of the GH/IGF-I pathway, is one of the most well-studied mechanisms and, perhaps, a critical determinant of life span. The free radical theory of aging proposes that endogenously generated ROS cause aging through damage to DNA, proteins, and lipids ***(80, 81)***. Numerous reports have documented the effects of GH and IGF-I on oxidative metabolism. Growth hormone is an anabolic factor that increases cellular metabolism. Increased metabolic activity (glucose oxidation and oxygen consumption) leads to increased oxidative phosphorylation and increased production of ROS as by-products of metabolism. Rollo and coworkers ***(82)*** showed that GH overexpression increased superoxide dismutase (SOD) radicals and oxidative damage to membrane lipids (lipid peroxidation). Tissues from mice with elevated plasma GH levels exhibit significantly reduced levels of antioxidative enzymes including SOD, catalase, and glutathione peroxidase (GPX) ***(83–85)***. In addition, direct effects of GH and IGF-I in vitro strongly support the in vivo data showing that these two hormones directly down regulate these enzymes in hepatocytes ***(86)***. Supporting this work, GH administration to GH-deficient Ames dwarf mice down regulates catalase, GPX, and SOD in both young and adult animals ***(87)***.

In contrast to the findings observed when GH is in excess, several reports demonstrate enhanced defense capacity of this system with GH deficiency. Ames dwarf mice exhibit elevated levels of catalase, GPX, SOD, and glutathione (GSH) in multiple tissues across their life span (Brown-Borg, unpublished data) ***(83, 84, 88)***. The thiol-containing proteins, metallothionein and GSH, are nonenzymatic antioxidant molecules exhibiting ROS scavenging abilities; their levels are elevated in tissues of Ames dwarf mice ***(9, 89)***. The amino acid pathway supporting GSH metabolism, methionine, is also highly upregulated in the Ames mouse ***(90–92)***.

Phenotypically identical Snell dwarf mice also exhibit an enhanced antioxidative defense capacity. Skin-derived fibroblasts from Snell mice are more resistant to multiple forms of cellular stress including percent increases in LD50 (lethal dose, 50%) values following exposure to UV light (45%), $H_2O_2$ (147%), paraquat (53%), cadmium (180%), and heat (102%) ***(93)***. These studies, along with others, indicate an overall increase in stress resistance to both oxidative and nonoxidative insults ***(94)***. Dwarf mice challenged with an inhibitor of succinate dehydrogenase (mitochondrial complex II), which caused increased free radical generation in tissues ***(95, 96)***, managed this oxidative stress differently than did the wild-type control mice ***(97)***. Although antioxidative defense enzymes have not been systematically evaluated in the Snell dwarf, an overall enhancement of this system is probably responsible for increased resistance to oxidative insult, as found in phenotypically identical Ames dwarf mice. Ames mice showed similar resistance to these cellular stressors (UV, 43%; $H_2O_2$, 79%; cadmium, 95%) as did GHRKO mice (UV, 194%; $H_2O_2$, 108%; paraquat, 47%) ***(94)***. The IGF-IR knockdown mice are also resistant to oxidative stress ***(28)*** as are mice that overexpress the protein klotho ***(31)***.

The GHRKO animals differ from Ames mice with regard to levels of the antioxidative enzymes catalase and GPX ***(98)***; they exhibit far less enhancement of GPX and no increases in catalase. We have new evidence showing that aspects of GSH metabolism are elevated but to a lower degree than in Ames mice (possibly reflecting the difference in GH signaling) ***(99)***.

Mitochondrial hydrogen peroxide production (liver) is significantly lower in Ames dwarf mice, likely indicating decreased metabolic activity in the absence of GH and thyroid hormone ***(100)***. The reduced ROS and elevated antioxidative capacity of dwarf mice lead to less nuclear DNA, mitochondrial DNA, and protein oxidative damage in several tissues ***(100, 101)***. Additionally, recent evidence reported by Choksi and coworkers ***(102)*** shows that Ames mice have lower levels of isoprostanes (indicative of lipid peroxidation) in both serum and liver, which suggests a lower level of oxidative stress. Functionality of the enhanced antioxidative capacity is verified in studies showing that Ames dwarf and IGF-IR heterozygous mice outsurvive their wild-type counterparts following paraquat administration ***(28, 103)***; in contrast, GHRKO mice either show no difference or succumb earlier than wild-type mice. Taken together, these studies suggest that low to normal plasma GH levels are consistent with resistance but that high levels suppress mechanisms that counter oxidative stress and support the concept that GH and IGF-I signaling pathways are intimately involved in this system.

Gene expression analysis supports evidence for enhanced stress resistance in Ames dwarf mice. Several genes involved in both phase I and II xenobiotic metabolism were found to be elevated in dwarf mice ***(104)***. Significantly enhanced activity of glutathione S-transferase has been reported in Ames mice ***(90)*** as have other components of the GSH metabolic pathway. These findings indicate that the Ames dwarf mouse exhibits characteristics that lead to an enhanced ability to counter genotoxic and metabolic insults.

Regarding other factors involved in stress resistance, Ames mice also exhibit greater heat shock protein levels and elevated levels of methionine sulfoxide reductase, an enzyme involved in protein repair ***(105)***. Dwarf mice and rats have been shown to resist cancer development following administration of a chemical carcinogen ***(106, 107)*** and exhibit a reduction in growth of transplanted tumors ***(108)***. Spontaneous tumor incidence is delayed and the severity is reduced in the dwarf mice ***(16, 109)***. Additionally, in both Midi and IGF-I deficient mice, tumor growth is reduced relative to that in control mice (Sell, personal communication) ***(110)***. These data make intuitive sense because GH and IGF-I are anabolic hormones, and as such, deficiencies in these hormones lead to a decreased propensity to develop tumors. It has been proposed that stress resistance is coordinately upregulated (heat shock proteins, antioxidants, detoxification systems, metal chelators, and repair systems) and that this increase results in multistress resistance to different stressors ***(45, 111, 112)***. Indeed, our studies as well as those by Murakami ***(93)*** and Salmon ***(94)*** show that cells from long-living mice exhibit enhanced defense mechanisms and are resistant to multiple forms of cellular stress.

## 7.4 Premature or Accelerated Aging

The longevity dividends are supported by evidence of delayed or decelerated aging in several of these GH mutants, including delayed sexual maturation, decreased tumor development, reduced tumor incidence, less osteoarthritis, and less age-dependent collagen cross-linking than in wild-type mice ***(16, 109, 113)***. Enhanced antioxidative defenses, lower ROS generation, and less oxidative damage also contribute to delays in age-related pathologic processes. Finally, evidence suggests that GH deficiency is associated with maintenance of cognitive function. Ames dwarf mice do not exhibit the age-related decline in cognitive function and behavior that is observed in wild-type control mice ***(114)***. Enhanced neurogenesis and elevated hippocampal IGF-I may explain the maintenance of cognitive activity in GH-deficient dwarf mice ***(115)***. Moreover, a recent report shows that hippocampal tissue of Ames dwarf mice also resists beta amyloid toxicity, evidence of enhanced defense ***(116)***.

In general, it appears that the degree of life-span extension is associated with the degree of both hormone deficiency and background strain, among other factors. Several other notable lines of study support the evidence that the somatotropic axis regulates life span. First, mice expressing GH transgenes are characterized by high plasma GH levels, increased body weights and lengths, multiple signs of premature aging (glomerulosclerosis, glomerulonephritis, mammary and liver tumors, early reproductive senescence, scoliosis, astrogliosis), and life spans half that of wild-type siblings (12 months; Bartke and Ikeno, unpublished) ***(42, 56, 57, 117–119)***. These data suggest that pharmacological levels of circulating GH lead to early onset of age-related pathologic changes in rodents. Second, overexpression of IGF-II in smooth muscle cells of mice shortens life span significantly ***(120)***. Third, high-dose GH treatment in rats has also proved to be toxic ***(121)***. Therefore, GH and IGF-I exert significant control over physiological processes that in turn affect aging.

## 7.5 Conclusions

The naturally occurring decline in plasma GH levels with age and the concomitant decrease in IGF-I that occurs in mammals are likely protective mechanisms to decrease metabolic activity and cellular division. Elevated levels of either GH or IGF-I throughout life contribute to the pathological changes associated with aging such as increased collagen cross-linking, osteoarthritis, immune system dysfunction, insulin resistance, oxidative damage, sensitivity to stress, and cancer. Most reports on hormones and aging in other species including nematodes and flies directly support the evidence in mammals. Some investigators have proposed that during evolution, the common GH/IGF/insulin pathway diverged into two, one to regulate cell division and growth and the other to control metabolism and partitioning of energy resources ***(122, 123)***. In nematodes, flies, and mammals, these metabolic pathways regulate energy, reproductive activity, and stress responses such that when food is abundant, growth, sexual maturation, and reproduction dominate. When food is scarce, resources are used to favor survival and directed away from growth and reproduction to increase stress resistance and repair processes leading to delayed aging and longevity. Overall, significant evolutionary evidence implicates the endocrine system, and the somatotropic axis in particular, as a major regulator of aging and life span.

## References


1. Mulinos M, Pomerantz, L. Psuedo-hypophysectomy, a condition resembling hypophysectomy produced by malnutrition. J Nutr 1940;19:493–500.
2. Everitt AV, Cavanagh LM. The ageing process in the hypophysectiomised rat. Gerontologia 1965;11:198–207.
3. Everitt AV, Porter B. Nutrition and aging. Springfield, IL: Charles C Thomas, 1976.
4. Everitt AV, Seedsman NJ, Jones F. The effects of hypophysectomy and continuous food restriction, begun at ages 70 and 400 days, on collagen aging, proteinuria, incidence of pathology and longevity in the male rat. Mech Ageing Dev 1980;12:161–72.
5. Powers RW, III, Harrison DE, Flurkey K. Pituitary removal in adult mice increases life span. Mech Ageing Dev 2006;127:658–9.
6. Corpas E, Harman SM, Blackman MR. Human growth hormone and human aging. Endocr Rev 1993;14:20–39.
7. Sonntag W, Hylka VW, Meites J. Impaired ability of old male rats to secrete growth hormone in vivo but not in vitro in response to hpGRF(1–44). Endocrinology 1983;113:2305–7.
8. Rudman D, Kutner MH, Rogers CM, Lubin MF, Fleming GA, Bain RP. Impaired growth hormone secretion in the adult population: relation to age and adiposity. J Clin Invest 1981;67:1361–9.
9. Brown-Borg HM, Borg KE, Meliska CJ, Bartke A. Dwarf mice and the ageing process. Nature 1996;384:33.
10. Bartke A. Genetic models in the study of anterior pituitary hormones. Boca Raton: CRC Press, 1979.
11. Sornson MW, Wu W, Dasen JS, Flynn SE, Norman DJ, O'Connell SM, Gukovsky I, Carriére C, Ryan AK, Miller AP, Zuo L, Gleiberman AS, Anderson B, Beamer WG, Rosenfeld MG. Pituitary lineage determination by the Prophet of Pit-1 homeodomain factor defective in Ames dwarfism. Nature 1996;384:327–33.
12. Chandrashekar V, Bartke A. Induction of endogenous insulin-like growth factor-I secretion alters the hypothalamic-pituitary-testicular function in growth hormone-deficient adult dwarf mice. Biol Reprod 1993;48:544–51.
13. Bartke A, Wright JC, Mattison JA, Ingram DK, Miller RA, Roth GS. Extending the lifespan of long-lived mice. Nature 2001;414:412.
14. Bartke A. Histology of the anterior hypophysis, thyroid and gonads of two types of dwarf mice. Anat Rec 1964;149:225–35.
15. Li S, Crenshaw EB, III, Rawson EJ, Simmons DM, Swanson LW, Rosenfeld MG. Dwarf locus mutants lacking three pituitary cell types result from mutations in the POU-domain gene pit-1. Nature 1990;347:528–33.
16. Flurkey K, Papaconstantinou J, Miller RA, Harrison DE. Lifespan extension and delayed immune and collagen aging in mutant mice with defects in growth hormone production. Proc Natl Acad Sci U S A 2001;98:6736–41.
17. Vergara M, Smith-Wheelock M, Harper JM, Sigler R, Miller RA. Hormone-treated snell dwarf mice regain fertility but remain long lived and disease resistant. J Gerontol 2004;59:1244–50.
18. Zhou Y, Xu BC, Maheshwari HG, He L, Reed M, Lozykowski M, Okada S, Wagner TE, Cataldo LA, Coschigano K, Baumann G, Kopchick JJ. A mammalian model for Laron syndrome produced by targeted disruption of the mouse growth hormone receptor/binding protein gene (the Laron mouse). Proc Natl Acad Sci U S A 1997;94:13215–20.
19. Coschigano KT, Clemmons D, Bellush LL, Kopchick JJ. Assessment of growth parameters and life span of GHR/BP gene-disrupted mice. Endocrinology 2000;141:2608–13.
20. Bartke A, Chandrashekar V, Dominici F, et al. Insulin-like growth factor 1 (IGF-1) and aging: controversies and new insights. Biogerontology 2003;4:1–8.
21. Eicher E, Beamer WG. Inherited ateliotic dwarfism in mice. Characteristics of mutation, little, on chromosome 6. J Hered 1976;67:87–91.

22. Godfrey P, Rahal JO, Beamer WG, Copeland NG, Jenkins NA, Mayo KE. GHRH receptor of little mice contains a missense mutation in the extracellular domain that disrupts receptor function. Nat Genet 1993;4:227–32.
23. Lin SC, Lin CR, Gukovsky I, Lusis AJ, Sawchenko PE, Rosenfeld MG. Molecular basis of the little mouse phenotype and implications for cell type-specific growth. Nature 1993;364:208–13.
24. Chen WY, White ME, Wagner TE, Kopchick JJ. Functional antagonism between endogenous mouse growth hormone (GH) and a GH analog results in dwarf transgenic mice. Endocrinology 1991;129:1402–8.
25. Liu J, LeRoith D. Insulin-like growth factor I is essential for postnatal growth in response to growth hormone. Endocrinology 1999;140:5178–84.
26. Liu JP, Baker J, Perkins AS, Robertson EJ, Efstratiadis A. Mice carrying null mutations of the genes encoding insulin-like growth factor I (Igf-1) and type 1 IGF receptor (Igf1r). Cell 1993;75:59–72.
27. Powell-Braxton L, Hollingshead P, Warburton C, Dowd M, Pitts-Meek S, Dalton D, Gillett H, Stewart TA. IGF-1 is required for normal embryonic growth in mice. Genes Dev 1996;7:2609–17.
28. Holzenberger M, Dupont J, Ducos B, Leneuve P, Geloen A, Even PC, Cervera P, Le Bouc Y IGF-1 receptor regulates lifespan and resistance to oxidative stress in mice. Nature 2003;421:182–7.
29. Yakar S, Liu JL, Stannard B, et al. Normal growth and development in the absence of hepatic insulin-like growth factor I. Proc Natl Acad Sci U S A 1999;96:7324–9.
30. Yakar S, Liu JL, Fernandez AM, Wu Y, Schally AV, Frystyk J, Chernausek SD, Mejia W, LeRoith D. Liver-specific igf-1 gene deletion leads to muscle insulin insensitivity. Diabetes 2001;50:1110–8.
31. Kurosu H, Yamamoto M, Clark JD, Pastor JV, Nandi A, Gurnani P, McGuinness OP, Chikuda H, Yamaguchi M, Takayama Y, Herz J, Kahn CR, Rosenblatt KP, Kuro-o M. Suppression of aging in mice by the hormone Klotho. Science 2005;309:1829–33.
32. Eicher EM, Beamer WG. Inherited ateliotic dwarfism in mice. Characteristics of mutation, little, on chromosome 6. J Hered 1976;67:87–91.
33. Shimokawa I, Higami Y, Utsuyama M, et al. Life span extension by reduction in growth hormone-insulin-like growth factor-1 axis in a transgenic rat model. Am J Pathol 2002;160:2259–65.
34. Charlton HM, Clark RG, Robinson IC, et al. Growth hormone-deficient dwarfism in the rat: a new mutation. J Endocrinol 1988;119:51–8.
35. Yakar S, Setser J, Zhao H, Stannard B, Haluzik M, Glatt V, Bouxsein ML, Kopchick JJ, LeRoith D. Inhibition of growth hormone action improves insulin sensitivity in liver IGF-1-deficient mice. J Clin Invest 2004;113:96–105.
36. Patronek GJ, Waters DJ, Glickman LT. Comparative longevity of pet dogs and humans: implications for gerontology research. J Gerontol 1997;52:B171–8.
37. Samaras TT, Elrick H, Storms LH. Is height related to longevity? Life Sci 2003;72:1781–802.
38. Comfort A. The lifespan of animals. Sci Am1961;205:108–19.
39. Roberts R. The lifetime growth and reproduction of selected strains of mice. Heredity 1961;16:369–81.
40. Duffy P, Feuers RJ, Hart RW. Effect of chronic caloric restriction on the circadian regulation of physiological and behavioral variables in old male B6C3F1 mice. Chronobiol Int 1990;7:291–303.
41. Shea BT, Hammer RE, Brinster RL. Growth allometry of the organs in giant transgenic mice. Endocrinology 1987;121:1924–30.
42. Wanke R, Wolf E, Hermanns W, Folger S, Buchmuller T, Brem G. The GH-transgenic mouse as an experimental model for growth research: clinical and pathological studies. Horm Res 1992;37 (Suppl 3):74–87.

43. Rollo CDKL, Wylie B, D'Souza S. The growth hormone axis, feeding, and central allocative regulation: Lessons from giant transgenic growth hormone mice. Can J Zool 1999;77:1861–73.
44. de Magalhaes JP, Cabral JA, Magalhaes D. The influence of genes on the aging process of mice: a statistical assessment of the genetics of aging. Genetics 2005;169:265–74.
45. Rollo CD. Growth negatively impacts the life span of mammals. Evol Dev 2002;4:55–61.
46. Baker J, Hardy MP, Zhou J, Bondy C, Lupu F, Bellve AR, Efstratiadis A. Effects of an Igf1 gene null mutation on mouse reproduction. Mol Endocrinol 1996;10:903–18.
47. Wang GM, O'Shaughnessy PJ, Chubb C, Robaire B, Hardy MP. Effects of insulin-like growth factor I on steroidogenic enzyme expression levels in mouse Leydig cells. Endocrinology 2003;144:4058–5064.
48. Bartke A. Delayed aging in Ames dwarf mice. Relationships to endocrine function and body size. Results Probl Cell Differ 2000;29:181–202.
49. Chubb C. Sexual behavior and fertility of little mice. Biol Reprod 1987;37:564–9.
50. Gravance CG, Breier BH, Vickers MH, Casey PJ. Impaired sperm characteristics in postpubertal growth-hormone-deficient dwarf (dw/dw) rats. Anim Reprod Sci 1997;49:71–6.
51. Vickers MH, Casey PJ, Champion ZJ, Gravance CG, Breier BH. IGF-I treatment increases motility and improves morphology of immature spermatozoa in the GH-deficient dwarf (dw/dw) rat. Growth Horm IGF Res 1999;9:236–40.
52. Weindruch R, Sohal RS. Seminars in medicine of the Beth Israel Deaconess Medical Center. Caloric intake and aging. N Engl J Med 1997;337:986–94.
53. Meites J. Anti-ageing interventions and their neuroendocrine aspects in mammals. J Reprod Fertil 1993;46:1–9.
54. Holehan AM, Merry BJ. The control of puberty in the dietary restricted female rat. Mech Ageing Dev 1985;32:179–91.
55. Chandrashekar V, Bartke A, Wagner TE. Endogenous human growth hormone (GH) modulates the effect of gonadotropin-releasing hormone on pituitary function and the gonadotropin response to the negative feedback effect of testosterone in adult male transgenic mice bearing human GH gene. Endocrinology 1988;123:2717–22.
56. Bartke A, Cecim M, Tang K, Steger RW, Chandrashekar V, Turyn D. Neuroendocrine and reproductive consequences of overexpression of growth hormone in transgenic mice. Proc Soc Exp Biol Med 1994;206:345–59.
57. Steger RW, Bartke A, Cecim M. Premature ageing in transgenic mice expressing different growth hormone genes. J Reprod Fertil Suppl. 1993;46:61–75.
58. Naar EM, Bartke A, Majumdar SS, Buonomo FC, Yun JS, Wagner TE. Fertility of transgenic female mice expressing bovine growth hormone or human growth hormone variant genes. Biol Reprod 1991;45:178–87.
59. Chandrashekar V, Zaczek D, Bartke A. The consequences of altered somatotropic system on reproduction. Biol Reprod 2004;71:17–27.
60. Balbis A, Bartke A, Turyn D. Overexpression of bovine growth hormone in transgenic mice is associated with changes in hepatic insulin receptors and in their kinase activity. Life Sci 1996;59:1363–71.
61. Dominici FP, Balbis A, Bartke A, Turyn D. Role of hyperinsulinemia on hepatic insulin receptor concentration and autophosphorylation in the presence of high growth hormone levels in transgenic mice overexpressing growth hormone gene. J Endocrinol 1998;159:15–25.
62. Dominici FP, Arostegui Diaz G, Bartke A, Kopchick JJ, Turyn D. Compensatory alterations of insulin signal transduction in liver of growth hormone receptor knockout mice. J Endocrinol 2000;166:579–90.
63. Dominici FP, Argentino DP, Bartke A, Turyn D. The dwarf mutation decreases high dose insulin responses in skeletal muscle, the opposite of effects in liver. Mech Ageing Dev 2003;124:819–27.
64. Borg KE, Brown-Borg HM, Bartke A. Assessment of the primary adrenal cortical and pancreatic hormone basal levels in relation to plasma glucose and age in the unstressed Ames dwarf mouse. Proc Soc Exp Biol Med 1995;210:126–33.

65. Barzilai N, Banerjee S, Hawkins M, Chen W, Rossetti L. Caloric restriction reverses hepatic insulin resistance in aging rats by decreasing visceral fat. J Clin Invest 1998;101:1353–61.
66. Barzilai N, She L, Liu BQ, et al. Surgical removal of visceral fat reverses hepatic insulin resistance. Diabetes 1999;48:94–8.
67. Hauck SJ, Hunter WS, Danilovich N, Kopchick JJ, Bartke A. Reduced levels of thyroid hormones, insulin, and glucose, and lower body core temperature in the growth hormone receptor/binding protein knockout mouse. Exp Biol Med (Maywood) 2001;226:552–8.
68. Dominici FP, Hauck S, Argentino DP, Bartke A, Turyn D. Increased insulin sensitivity and upregulation of insulin receptor, insulin receptor substrate (IRS)-1 and IRS-2 in liver of Ames dwarf mice. J Endocrinol 2002;173:81–94.
69. Brooks NL, Trent CM, Raetzsch CF, Flurkey K, Boysen G, Perfetti MT, Jeong Y-C, Klebanov S, Patel KB, Khodush VR, Kupper LL, Carling D, Swenberg JA, Harrison DE, Combs TP. Low utilization of circulating glucose after food withdrawal in snell dwarf mice. J Biol Chem 2007;282:35069–77.
70. Parsons JA, Bartke A, Sorenson RL. Number and size of islets of Langerhans in pregnant, human growth hormone-expressing transgenic, and pituitary dwarf mice: Effect of lactogenic hormones. Endocrinology 1995;136:2013–21.
71. Yu R, Yakar S, Liu YL, et al. Liver-specific IGF-I gene deficient mice exhibit accelerated diabetes in response to streptozotocin, associated with early onset of insulin resistance. Mol Cell Endocrinol 2003;204:31–42.
72. Reiser KM. Nonenzymatic glycation of collagen in aging and diabetes. Proc Soc Exp Biol Med 1998;218:23–37.
73. Monnier VM. Toward a Maillard reaction theory of aging. Prog Clin Biol Res 1989;304:1–22.
74. Facchini FS, Hua N, Abbasi F, Reaven GM. Insulin resistance as a predictor of age-related diseases. J Clin Endocrinol Metab 2001;86:3574–8.
75. Bluher M, Michael MD, Peroni OD, et al. Adipose tissue selective insulin receptor knockout protects against obesity and obesity-related glucose intolerance. Dev Cell 2002;3:25–38.
76. Bluher M, Kahn BB, Kahn CR. Extended longevity in mice lacking the insulin receptor in adipose tissue. Science 2003;299:572–4.
77. Paolisso G, Gambardella A, Ammendola S, D'Amore A, Balbi V, Varricchio M, D'Onofrio F. Glucose tolerance and insulin action in healthy centenarians. Am J Physiol 1996;270(5 Pt 1):E890–E894.
78. Paolisso G, Barbieri M, Rizzo MR, et al. Low insulin resistance and preserved beta-cell function contribute to human longevity but are not associated with TH-INS genes. Exp Gerontol 2001;37:149–56.
79. Brown-Borg HM. Hormonal regulation of longevity in mammals. Ageing Res Rev 2007;6:28–45.
80. Harman D. Aging: A theory based on free radical and radiation chemistry. J Gerontol 1956;11:298–300.
81. Harman D. Free radicals in aging. Mol Cell Biochem 1988;84:155–61.
82. Rollo CD, Sawada M. Accelerated aging of giant transgenic mice is associated with elevated free radical processes. Can J Zool 1996;74:606–20.
83. Brown-Borg HM, Bode AM, Bartke A. Antioxidative mechanisms and plasma growth hormone levels: Potential relationship in the aging process. Endocrine 1999;11:41–8.
84. Brown-Borg HM, Rakoczy SG. Catalase expression in delayed and premature aging mouse models. Exp Gerontol 2000;35:199–212.
85. Hauck SJ, Bartke A. Free radical defenses in the liver and kidney of human growth hormone transgenic mice: Possible mechanisms of early mortality. J Gerontol 2001;56:B153–B162.
86. Brown-Borg HM, Rakoczy SG, Romanick MA, Kennedy MA. Effects of growth hormone and insulin-like growth factor-1 on hepatocyte antioxidative enzymes. Exp Biol Med (Maywood) 2002;227:94–104.
87. Brown-Borg HM, Rakoczy SG. Growth hormone administration to long-living dwarf mice alters multiple components of the antioxidative defense system. Mech Ageing Dev 2003;124:1013–24.

88. Hauck SJ, Bartke A. Effects of growth hormone on hypothalamic catalase and Cu/Zn superoxide dismutase. Free Radic Biol Med 2000;28:970–8.
89. Meyer M, Swinscoe JC, Brown-Borg HM, Carlson EC. Increased glomerular metallothionein accompanies reduced glomerular basement membrane thickening in the Ames dwarf model of delayed aging. Exp Biol 2003:217.1.
90. Brown-Borg HM, Rakoczy SG. Glutathione metabolism in long-living Ames dwarf mice. Exp Gerontol 2005;40:115–20.
91. Uthus EO, Brown-Borg HM. Altered methionine metabolism in long living Ames dwarf mice. Exp Gerontol 2003;38:491–8.
92. Uthus EO, Brown-Borg HM. Methionine flux to transsulfuration is enhanced in the long living Ames dwarf mouse. Mech Ageing Dev 2006;127:444–50.
93. Murakami S, Salmon A, Miller RA. Multiplex stress resistance in cells from long-lived dwarf mice. FASEB J 2003;17:1565–6.
94. Salmon AB, Murakami S, Bartke A, Kopchick J, Yasumura K, Miller RA. Fibroblast cell lines from young adult mice of long-lived mutant strains are resistant to multiple forms of stress. Am J Physiol Endocrinol Metab 2005;289:E23–E29.
95. Coles CJ, Edmondson DE, Singer TP. Inactivation of succinate dehydrogenase by 3-nitropropionate. J Biol Chem 1979;254:5161–7.
96. Fu YT, He FS, Zhang SL, Zhang JS. Lipid peroxidation in rats intoxicated with 3-nitropropionic acid. Toxicon 1995;33:327–31.
97. Madsen MA, Hsieh CC, Boylston WH, Flurkey K, Harrison D, Papaconstantinou J. Altered oxidative stress response of the long-lived Snell dwarf mouse. Biochem Biophys Res Commun 2004;318:998–1005.
98. Hauck SJ, Aaron JM, Wright C, Kopchick JJ, Bartke A. Antioxidant enzymes, free-radical damage, and response to paraquat in liver and kidney of long-living growth hormone receptor/binding protein gene-disrupted mice. Horm Metab Res 2002;34:481–6.
99. Brown-Borg HM, Rakoczy SG, Sharma S, Bartke A. Long-living growth hormone receptor knockout mice: Potential mechanisms of altered stress resistance. Exp Gerontol 2009;44:10–9.
100. Brown-Borg HM, Johnson WT, Rakoczy SG, Kennedy MA, Romanick MA. Mitochondrial oxidant production and oxidative damage in Ames dwarf mice. J Am Aging Assoc 2001;24:85–96.
101. Sanz A, Barja G. Long-lived Ames dwarf mice: Oxidative damage to mitochondrial DNA in heart and brain. J Am Aging Assoc 2002;25:119–22.
102. Roberts LJ, II, DeFord JH, Rabek JP, Papaconstantinou J. Lower levels of F2-isoprostanes in serum and livers of long-lived Ames dwarf mice. Biochem BiophysRes Commun 2007;364:761–4.
103. Bartke A, Brown-Borg, HM, Kinney, B, Mattison, J, Wright, C, Hauck S, Coschigano K, Kopchick JJ. Growth hormone and aging. J Am Aging Assoc 2000;23:219–25.
104. Tsuchiya T, Dhahbi JM, Cui X, Mote PL, Bartke A, Spindler SR. Additive regulation of hepatic gene expression by dwarfism and caloric restriction. Physiol Genomics 2004;17:307–15.
105. Brown-Borg HM. Aging and life span. Adv Exp Med Biol 2005;567:259–83.
106. Bielschowsky F, Bielschowsky M. Carcinogenesis in the pituitary of dwarf mouse. The response to dimethylbenzanthracene applied to the skin. Br J Cancer 1961;15:257–62.
107. Ramsey MM, Ingram RL, Cashion AB, et al. Growth hormone-deficient dwarf animals are resistant to dimethylbenzanthracine (DMBA)-induced mammary carcinogenesis. Endocrinology 2002;143:4139–42.
108. Rennels EG, Anigstein DM, Anigstein L. A cumulative study of the growth of sarcoma 180 in anterior pituitary dwarf mice. Tex Rep Biol Med 1965;23:776–81.
109. Ikeno Y, Bronson RT, Hubbard GB, Lee S, Bartke A. Delayed occurrence of fatal neoplastic diseases in ames dwarf mice: correlation to extended longevity. J Gerontol 2003;58:291–6.
110. Yang XF, Beamer WG, Huynh H, Pollak M. Reduced growth of human breast cancer xenografts in hosts homozygous for the lit mutation. Cancer Res 1996;56:1509–11.

111. Jazwinski SM. Longevity, genes, and aging. Science 1996;273:54–9.
112. Martin GM, Austad SN, Johnson TE. Genetic analysis of ageing: role of oxidative damage and environmental stresses. Nat Genet 1996;13:25–34.
113. Silberberg R. Articular aging and osteoarthrosis in dwarf mice. Pathol Microbiol (Basel) 1972;38:417–30.
114. Kinney BA, Meliska CJ, Steger RW, Bartke A. Evidence that Ames dwarf mice age differently from their normal siblings in behavioral and learning and memory parameters. Horm Behav 2001;39:277–84.
115. Sun LY, Evans MS, Hsieh J, Panici J, Bartke A. Increased neurogenesis in dentate gyrus of long-lived Ames dwarf mice. Endocrinology 2005;146:1138–44.
116. Schrag M, Sharma S, Brown-Borg H, Ghribi O. Hippocampus of Ames dwarf mice is resistant to beta-amyloid-induced tau hyperphosphorylation and changes in apoptosis-regulatory protein levels. Hippocampus 2008;18:239–44.
117. Doi T, Striker LJ, Quaife C, et al. Progressive glomerulosclerosis develops in transgenic mice chronically expressing growth hormone and growth hormone releasing factor but not in those expressing insulin-like growth factor-1. Am J Pathol 1988;131:398–403.
118. Quaife CJ, Mathews LS, Pinkert CA, Hammer RE, Brinster RL, Palmiter RD. Histopathology associated with elevated levels of growth hormone and insulin-like growth factor I in transgenic mice. Endocrinology 1989;124:40–8.
119. Miller DB, Bartke A, O'Callaghan JP. Increased glial fibrillary acidic protein (GFAP) levels in the brains of transgenic mice expressing the bovine growth hormone (bGH) gene. Exp Gerontol 1995;30:383–400.
120. Zaina S, Pettersson L, Thomsen AB, et al. Shortened life span, bradycardia, and hypotension in mice with targeted expression of an Igf2 transgene in smooth muscle cells. Endocrinology 2003;144:2695–703.
121. Groesbeck MD, Parlow AF, Daughaday WH. Stimulation of supranormal growth in prepubertal, adult plateaued, and hypophysectomized female rats by large doses of rat growth hormone: physiological effects and adverse consequences. Endocrinology 1987;120:1963–75.
122. Guarente L, Kenyon C. Genetic pathways that regulate ageing in model organisms. Nature 2000;408:255–62.
123. Finch CE, Ruvkun G. The genetics of aging. Annu Rev Genomics Hum Genet 2001;2:435–62.

# Part V
# Comparative Biology of Aging

# Chapter 8
# Exploiting Natural Variation in Life Span to Evaluate Mechanisms of Aging

**Rochelle Buffenstein**

**Abstract** A 40,000-fold variation exists in maximum longevity across the animal kingdom. Even among mammals, naturally occurring differences in maximum life span among similar-sized species far exceed experimental life-span extension induced by genetic manipulations and/or caloric restriction. Elucidating mechanisms of different aging rates and of concomitant disparate longevity among different species of similar body composition, biochemistry, and physiology may provide new insights into aging and may also be used to test the ubiquity of findings reported with traditional models. As such, studies employing a comparative approach to aging are poised to make pivotal inroads leading to understanding the mechanisms of aging.

**Keywords** Longevity • longevity quotient • bats • reptiles • mole-rats • oxidative stress

**Abbreviations** LQ: Longevity quotient; MLS: Maximum species life span

## 8.1 Introduction

Although death may not always be due to age-related causes, maximum species life span (MLS) is, nevertheless, considered an important species characteristic. Reported MLS varies more than 100-fold among mammals and 40,000-fold across the animal kingdom *(1)*. These naturally occurring differences in mammalian longevity are much greater than those that can be experimentally induced through caloric

R. Buffenstein
The Sam and Ann Barshop Institute for Longevity and Aging Studies and Department of Physiology, University of Texas Health Science Center at San Antonio,
San Antonio, TX, 78245, USA
e-mail: Buffenstein@uthscsa.edu

C. Sell et al. (eds.), *Life-Span Extension,* Aging Medicine,
DOI 10.1007/978-1-60327-507-1_8,

restriction or single-gene mutations ***(2)***. Understanding what mechanisms the evolutionary forces of nature use to create species with disparate longevity is a fundamental research focus in comparative aging research. Species differences in longevity must be encoded in the genome and imply that genotypic intrinsic mechanisms primarily determine aging rate. These mechanisms are present throughout life. As such, species differences in aging can be discerned in young and old individuals. The ability of the genome to evolve mechanisms that ensure longevity can, however, only be expressed when a species is protected from extrinsic factors (e.g., predation and climatic extremes). Exogenous factors (environmental stressors, e.g., toxic chemicals) may interact with genotype-dependent factors, either enhancing or diminishing their effects, and thereby also influence rates of aging ***(3)***. Although extrinsic factors may contribute to the aging process, they themselves are not determinants of maximum species life span. The combined effects of intrinsic determinants and extrinsic modulators may explain why various species or strains, maintained under similar conditions, age at different rates.

Every model organism studied in biogerontology has different strengths and weaknesses and can provide unique information relative to aging. For example, on the one hand, short-lived species such as worms, flies, fish, and mice may be effectively used in longitudinal studies to provide answers in response to experimental manipulation or life span extension effects of pharmaceutical agents within a relatively short period (see Chap. 11). These kinds of studies are impractical in long-living organisms. On the other hand, long-living organisms enable one to assess both evolutionary and proximate mechanisms that may have evolved for successful slow aging and prolonged health span (see Chap. 10). Studies examining differences in the physiology and cellular biology of species whose maximum life spans vary may provide insights into the intrinsic mechanisms that modulate the rate of age-related physiological decline. Understanding these mechanisms may provide important insights for enhancing health span rather than simply extending life span. Humans are inherently interested in and wish to emulate the mechanisms of successful aging that enhance health and vigor.

## 8.2 Relation Between MLS and Body Size

MLS lengthens in a predictable manner as species increase in size such that for every doubling of body mass in mammals, on average a 16% increase occurs in MLS (Fig. 8.1). Body mass can, however, explain only about 35% of the variation in mammalian MLS. MLS appears to be taxon specific, such that among mammals, cetaceans, primates, and bats have higher longevity quotients (LQs, i.e., live longer than predicted by size), whereas marsupials are shorter-lived (Fig. 8.2) ***(4, 5)***. Rodent longevity generally follows the expected allometric relationship. For its size, *Homo sapiens* is a long-living mammal, with an MLS (122.5 years) about five times longer than predicted by mass for terrestrial nonflying mammals. To date, we do not know why humans and a few other long-living mammals are outliers from

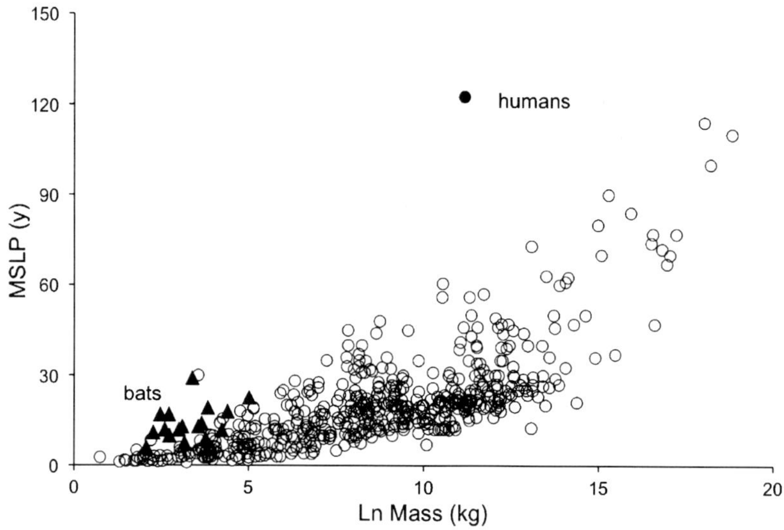


**Fig. 8.1** The allometric relationship between body size and maximum life span (MLS) for 500 nonvolant mammals. Data from the various orders generally fall close to the descriptor (MLS = M 0.21), notable exceptions are humans (*circles*) and bats (*triangles*)

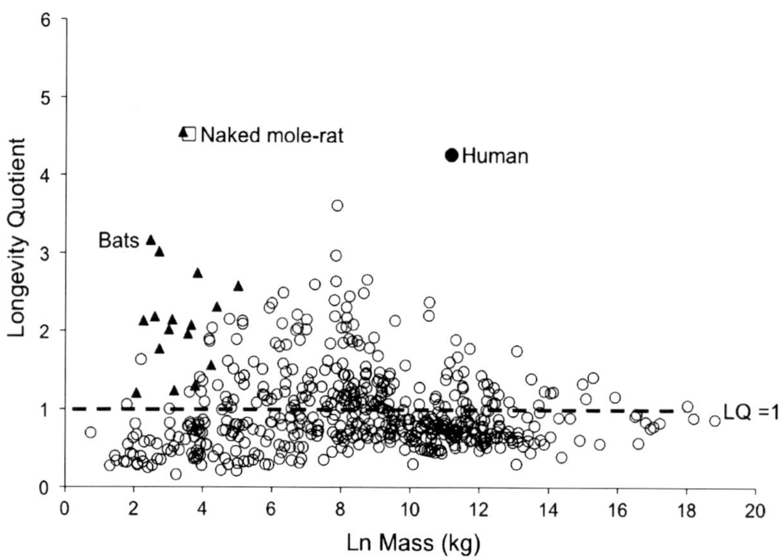


**Fig. 8.2** The longevity quotient [the ratio of observed maximum life span to that predicted by body mass using the equation of de Magalhaes *(4)*]. Although only nonvolant mammals were used in this equation, when it was used to determine the LQ of bats, bats all have high LQs, as do naked mole-rats; humans have exceptionally high LQs

this allometric relationship, nor do we understand the mechanisms that facilitate aging. Understanding endogenous causes and interspecific differences of this ubiquitous and inevitable process remains a key focus for biogerontologic studies.

## 8.3 Comparative Approach

Comparative studies exploiting differences in short-lived and long-lived organisms may reveal important insights into shared mechanisms of aging as well as highlight private mechanisms of aging *(6)*. The comparative biology approach can be used in two complementary ways. First, by determining how species differ at the molecular, cellular, and physiological levels, one can determine whether traits correlate with life span and then use that information to form testable hypotheses about the mechanisms that determine the rate of aging. Second, comparative biology draws attention to nontraditional model organisms, in particular those species that have evolved exceptional capabilities, including those that show unusually long maximal life spans. Studying organisms with unusual properties provides huge payoffs with respect to understanding biological phenomena. Two simple examples illustrate this point: Large simple axons in squid elucidated general mechanisms involved in neuronal action potentials whereas regulation of capillary action in frog skin, an important respiratory organ of frogs, earned the founding father of comparative biology, August Krogh, the Nobel Prize. He stated that "for every biological problem there is an animal species in which it is best studied" *(7)*. Clearly, even in biogerontology, unusual species should be viewed not as oddities but as unexplored resources. Comparative differences among species with disparate longevity provide a powerful source of putative mechanistic traits that can be further explored in depth; however, uncritical application may lead to numerous erroneous generalizations. This observation is especially true when comparisons are made between organisms with different complexities of biological organization and where specialized functional adaptations have evolved.

Two problems routinely plague comparative studies: The covariation of a specific trait with body mass is frequently ignored when interpreting findings, and phylogenetic relatedness between species may affect the statistical independence of data suites. It is an axiom of comparative biology that species with a close evolutionary relationship share more traits than more distantly related species, and comparative studies ignoring phylogeny may lead to pseudoreplication and spurious conclusions *(8)*.

## 8.4 Animal Models

Biogerontologists have converged on only a few model organisms (single-celled yeast, *Saccharomyces cerevisiae*; the nematode *Caenorhabditis elegans*; the fruit fly *Drosophila melanogaster;* and the laboratory mouse *Mus musculus*). More than

90% of all articles on nonhuman aging published in the last 20 years focus on these four divergent species, even though they represent a minute fraction of the animal kingdom. These four species have provided extremely valuable insights into putative regulators of longevity including the genetic, molecular, and biochemical bases and have contributed immensely to current understanding of aging processes.

Nontraditional model organisms provide an opportunity to test the generalizations drawn from traditional models and to extend studies on short-lived invertebrates to short-lived and long-lived vertebrates. Finch and Austad ***(9)*** reported that extremely long-lived organisms are found throughout the animal kingdom and include social insects (ants, bees, and wasps), crustacean bivalves (clams), fish (rockfish), reptiles (snakes), birds (parrots), and mammals (cetaceans, bats, and mole-rats). Not surprisingly, given the extended time demands of life-span studies in such animals as well as the difficulty of housing them, few studies involve these animals.

Organisms that live at least twice as long as expected from allometric studies (Fig. 8.2), such as bats and mole-rats as well as birds, fish, and social insects, are good candidates for discerning mechanisms used in slow aging ***(10, 11)***. Less can be gleaned from animals with LQs (ratio of reported MLS to that predicted by mass) less than one, because it is extremely difficult to discriminate the effects of accelerated aging from those of altered susceptibility to disease and inadequate husbandry of captive exotic species.

## 8.5 Insights from Comparative Studies

Most biogerontological studies involving nontraditional model organisms have focused predominantly on one proximate theory, namely, the oxidative stress theory of aging ***(12–17)***. Surprisingly, equivocal findings have been reported, leading one to question the causative vs. correlative role of oxidative stress in longevity. Many long-living rodents, reptiles, bats, and birds ***(10, 12–14, 18)*** have high levels of oxidative stress that are not commensurate with their longevity. Within just one taxonomic class, for example, bats or rodents (Fig. 8.3), longer-living species such as vampire bats and *Myotis* have higher oxidative damage levels than shorter-lived species that do not correlate with longevity ***(12, 17)*** (Hermes Lim, personal communication).

A strong relationship between species longevity and cellular resistance to oxidative insults has, nevertheless, been reported in a wide variety of organisms with disparate longevity ***(19–22)***. Cellular stress resistance extends to numerous other nonoxidative factors including heat, heavy metals that are not involved in redox reactions, chemotherapeutic agents, dietary alterations, and xenobiotics. Mechanisms include coordinated upregulation of features such as antioxidant defense systems, heat shock proteins, metal chelators, DNA and protein repair pathways, cell death and senescence induction, and protein degradation pathways. This disparate stress resistance among different species with disparate longevity reveals differential gene transcription or epigenetic imprinting. Cellular stress resistance is not only critically involved in aging processes, but it is also a critical component retarding the

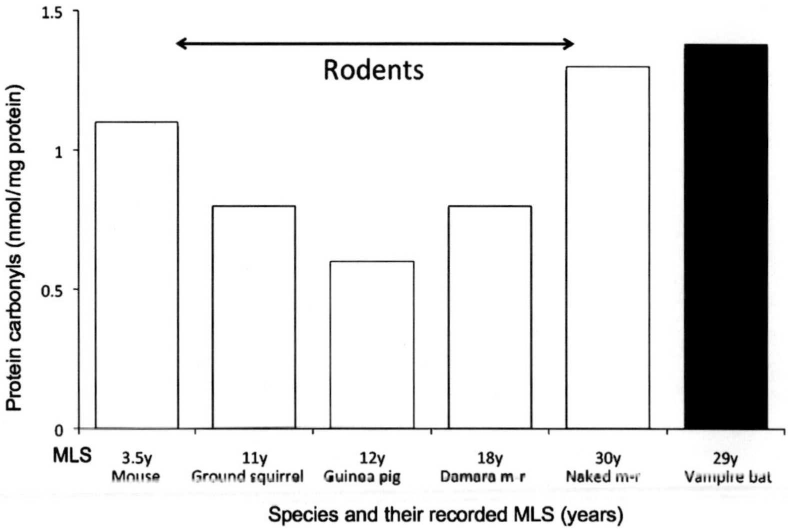


**Fig. 8.3** Protein carbonyls from five rodent species and one bat species with disparate maximum life-span (MLS; indicated in years (y) above the species) longevity. Note that no correlation exists between this marker of oxidative damage and maximum life span; indeed, young, long-living naked mole-rats and vampire bats have higher levels of protein carbonyl than do physiologically age-matched mice

onset and development of numerous age-related pathologic conditions including many cancers, neurodegenerative diseases, and atherosclerosis. Understanding mechanistic differences among species with different life-span potentials would provide pivotal insights into aging and extensive collateral benefits to numerous critical areas of health care. The challenge ahead is to determine what these are.

## 8.6 Conclusions

The use of traditional animal models has led to considerable progress in research on aging and continues to hold great promise for further advancing our knowledge of the aging process and potential intervention mechanisms. However, much more work is needed to identify novel model organisms for aging research. These organisms may provide new insights into successful aging and may also be used to test the ubiquity of findings reported with traditional models. The comparative biology of aging is poised to make pivotal inroads leading to understanding the mechanisms of aging.

**Acknowledgments** Funding from the NIH/NIA (AG 022891) is gratefully acknowledged.

## References


1. Finch CE. Longevity, senescence and the genome. Chicago: University of Chicago Press, 1990.
2. Hulbert AJ, Pamplona R, Buffenstein R, Buttemer WA. Life and death: Metabolic rate, membrane composition and lifespan of animals. Physiol Rev 2007;87:1175–213.
3. Ricklefs RE, Finch CE. Aging: A natural history. New York: Scientific American Library, HPHLP, 1995.
4. de Magalhaes JP, Costa J, Church GM. An analysis of the relationship between metabolism, developmental schedules, and longevity using phylogenetic independent contrasts. J Gerontol A Biol Sci Med Sci 2007;62:149–60.
5. Austad SN, Fischer KE. Mammalian aging, metabolism, and ecology: Evidence from bats and marsupials. J Gerontol 1991;46:B47–53.
6. Martin GM. Keynote lecture: An update on the what, why and how questions of ageing. Exp Gerontol 2006;41:460–3.
7. Krogh A. The progress of physiology. Science1929;70:200–4.
8. Speakman JR. Body size, energy metabolism and lifespan. J Exp Biol 2005;208:1717–30.
9. Finch CE, Austad SN. History and prospects: symposium on organisms with slow aging. Exp Gerontol 2001;36:593–7.
10. Buffenstein R. The naked mole-rat: A new long-living model for human aging research? J Gerontol 2005;60:1369–77.
11. Keller L, Jemielty S. Social insects as a model to study the molecular basis of ageing. Exp Gerontol 2006;41:553–6.
12. Brunet Rossinni AK. Testing the free radical theory of aging in bats. Ann N Y Acad Sci 2004;1019:506–8.
13. Costantini D, Cardinale M, Carere C. Oxidative damage and anti-oxidant capacity in two migratory bird species at a stop-over site. Comp Biochem Physiol C Toxicol Pharmacol 2007;144:363–71.
14. Furtado-Filho OV, Polcheira C, Machado DP, Mourão G, Hermes-Lima M. Selected oxidative stress markers in a South American crocodilian species. Comp Biochem Physiol C Toxicol Pharmacol 2007;146:241–54.
15. Lambert AJ, Boysen HM, Buckingham JA, et al. Low rates of hydrogen peroxide production by isolated heart mitochondria associate with long maximum lifespan in vertebrate homeotherms. Aging Cell 2007;6:607–18.
16. Robert KA, Brunet-Rossinni A, Bronikowski AM. Testing the 'free radical theory of aging' hypothesis: physiological differences in long-lived and short-lived colubrid snakes. Aging Cell 2007;6:395–404.
17. Wilhelm Filho D, Althoff SL, Dafré AL, Boveris A. Antioxidant defenses, longevity and ecophysiology of South American bats. Comp Biochem Physiol C Toxicol Pharmacol 2007;146:214–20.
18. Hamilton ML, Guo Z, Fuller CD, et al. A reliable assessment of 8-oxo-2-deoxyguanosine levels in nuclear and mitochondrial DNA using the sodium iodide method to isolate DNA. Nucleic Acids Res 2001;29:2117–26.
19. Kapahi P, Boulton ME, Kirkwood TB. Positive correlation between mammalian life span and cellular resistance to stress. Free Radic Biol Med 1999;26:495–500.
20. Salmon AB, Murakami S, Bartke A, Kopchick J, Yasumura K, Miller RA. Fibroblast cell lines from young adult mice of long-lived mutant strains are resistant to multiple forms of stress. Am J Physiol Endocrinol Metab 2005;289(1):E23–9.
21. Harper JM, Salmon AB, Leiser SF, Galecki AT, Miller RA. Skin-derived fibroblasts from long-lived species are resistant to some, but not all, lethal stresses and to the mitochondrial inhibitor rotenone. Aging Cell 2007;6:1–13.
22. Labinskyy N, Csiszar A, Orosz Z, et al. Comparison of endothelial function, $O_{2-}$* and H2O2 production, and vascular oxidative stress resistance between the longest-living rodent, the naked mole rat, and mice. Am J Physiol Heart Circ Physiol 2006;291:H2698–704.

# Chapter 9
# Slow Aging: Insights from an Exceptionally Long-Lived Rodent, the Naked Mole-Rat

**Rochelle Buffenstein and Yael H. Edrey**

**Abstract** As organisms age, one commonly notes a decline in vitality, fertility, and function with a concomitant increase in mortality risk. In short-lived animals, this decline is rapid, reflecting poor defense against aging. On the other hand, long-living organisms may show markedly attenuated rates of aging. Investigating how this is achieved may elucidate key mechanisms employed in slow or successful aging, characteristics we are interested in better understanding and even emulating. One such extraordinarily long-lived organism is the naked mole-rat. Naked mole-rats live in captivity an order of magnitude longer than similar-sized mice (>30 years). The common cause of death is still unknown and to date cancer has not been observed in these long-living rodents. Unlike the situation with most mammals, females continue to breed throughout their long lives and exhibit no decline in fertility well into their third decade. Only slight age-related changes are observed in all biochemical, physiological, and morphological characteristics studied to date. Clearly, these endogenous processes have evolved to dramatically extend healthy life span in this species, and typical age-associated acceleration in mortality risk that characterizes other mammalian species is attenuated. Studies addressing mechanisms of aging in this species have yielded surprising data: Naked mole-rat reproductive profiles are not typical of slow-aging K-selected animals and do not support the disposable soma theory of aging; short telomeres and low levels of telomerase in somatic tissue are in conflict with the telomere theory of aging; and high levels of oxidative damage diverge from those expected from the oxidative stress theory of aging. The challenge that lies ahead is to determine the mechanisms that facilitate the unusual profile

R. Buffenstein (✉)
The Sam and Ann Barshop Institute for Longevity and Aging Studies and the Department of Physiology, University of Texas Health Science Center at San Antonio, 15355 Lambda Dr STCBM 2.2, San Antonio, TX, 78245, USA
e-mail: Buffenstein@uthscsa.edu

Y.H. Edrey
The Sam and Ann Barshop Institute for Longevity and Aging Studies, University of Texas Health Science Center at San Antonio, 15355 Lambda Dr, STCBM 2.2, San Antonio, TX, 78245, USA

C. Sell et al. (eds.), *Life-Span Extension,* Aging Medicine,
DOI 10.1007/978-1-60327-507-1_9,

associated with slow aging and prolonged health span in this rodent, and to test the ubiquity of these mechanisms in other species. As such, the naked mole-rat will prove to be an important animal model with which to address successful aging.

**Keywords** Slow aging • maximum life span • oxidative stress • reproduction • *Heterocephalus glaber*

**Abbreviations** BMR: Basal metabolic rate; LEE: Lifetime energy expenditure; LQ: Longevity quotient; MLS: Maximum species life span; MLSP: Maximum life span potential; NO: Nitric oxide; ROS: Reactive oxygen species; TPI: Triosephosphate isomerase

## 9.1 Introduction

Maximum species life span (MLS) is an important species trait that increases as body size increases. Within rodents, life spans vary by an order of magnitude (Fig. 9.1). The shortest life span of a rodent is approximately 2 years, whereas the longest life span of a rodent, that of the naked mole-rat (Rodentia; Bathyergidae; *Heterocephalus glaber*, Rupell 1842; Fig. 9.2), is greater than 30 years. This life span is a new longevity record for this species and exceeds that previously reported by 2 years *(1)*. The new record holder is a female that was caught in the wild in June 1980 and

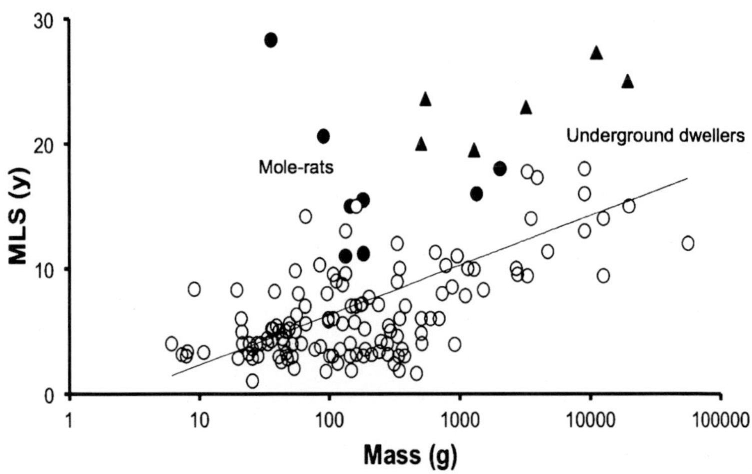


**Fig. 9.1** Maximum species life span (MLS) as a function of body mass for rodents. Please note that data from underground dwelling rodents (black triangles and black circles) generally lie above the descriptor and that the bathyergid mole-rats (*solid circles*) are particularly long-lived

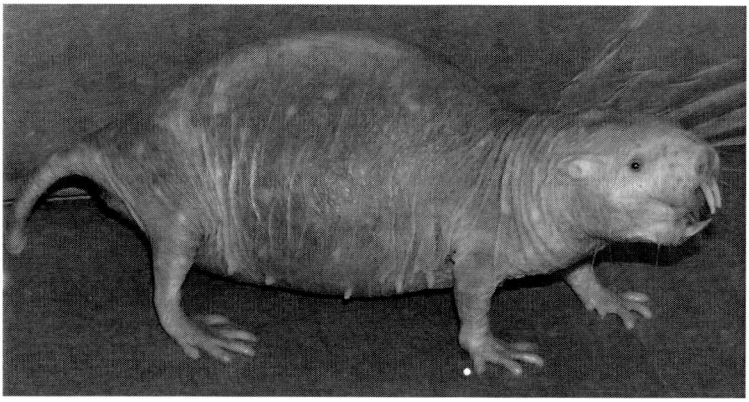

**Fig. 9.2** The naked mole-rat, a 15-year-old pregnant breeding female

already the dominant breeding female of the colony. Given her adult mass and breeding status upon capture, she would have had to have been at least 2 years old at capture. Although she was extremely frail, her death in May 2008 was not induced by disease but rather was due to accidental hypothermia. At the time of her death, she was, surprisingly, ovulating but had not successfully raised a litter in many years. Based upon her longevity record, she lived approximately five times longer than predicted by body size [Fig. 9.3; longevity quotient (LQ), using allometric equations of de Magalhães et al. *(2)*] and approximately 9-fold longer than laboratory mice (~3.5 years; LQ = 0.7). Although life in captivity is fraught with its own suite of physiologically stressful issues and restricted exercise, captive care removes many compounding factors affecting life span, such as predation and exposure to excessive temperatures, restricted water, and nutrient availability. MLS has a strong genetic foundation; MLS in captive animals may, therefore, more closely reflect phylogenetic traits and the cellular and molecular constraints of longevity.

Animals that acquire prolonged longevity generally have evolved in environments protected from extrinsic mortality. In unpredictable environments (e.g., arid and semi-arid, where food and water availability may be unpredictable), organisms produce as many offspring as quickly as possible, although mortality rates are often extremely high (r-selected); in safe and predictable habitats, fewer offspring are produced and more resources are invested in their long-term care (K-selected) with concomitant lower mortality rates (Table 9.1) *(4)*.

Subterranean animals, protected from both climatic extremes and predation, tend to live longer than above-ground-dwelling, similar-sized species (Fig. 9.1) *(5)*; flying mammals (e.g., bats) that rest in inaccessible localities (e.g., caves) or avoid land predators by flying are also extremely long-lived *(6)*, as are those vertebrates that present an impenetrable and/or armored façade when under attack (e.g., tortoises and porcupines). Similarly, colony members of eusocial insects (e.g., honey bees and ants) that are exposed to external stressors have substantially shorter life spans than those of their shielded “queens” *(7)*.

Extended longevity is also correlated with group or social living. Bats that live in large roosts, social primates, colony dwelling mole-rats, and eusocial insects all show prolonged longevity ***(5, 7–9)***. Enhanced fitness in these species may reflect communal protection from predation as well as the ability to modify environmental conditions by producing heat or acting as a larger single "unit" with concomitant changes in heat loss and/or metabolic rate associated with group living ***(10)***. Eusociality has evolved independently in several invertebrate groups as well as in subterranean bathyergid rodents, and both the eusocial insects and mole-rats exhibit extended longevity ***(11, 12)***. Living socially in large family units enhances inclusive fitness by kinship, cooperative care of young, and division of labor. This division of labor focuses the cost of reproduction on a few individuals and foraging costs on others. These features contribute to the model of socially induced longevity extension by increasing the survival of both young and reproductively active animals through intergenerational transfer of information, extended care, and complex social behavior associated with natural, sexual, and kin selection ***(5, 8)***.

Among rodents, naked mole-rats conspicuously stand out as being exceptionally long-lived, with an LQ that far exceeds that of any other rodent species (Fig. 9.3). Not only can we glean from this mouse-sized (~35 g) hystricognath species considerable insight into the various evolutionary theories of aging (alluded to above), but we may also be able to obtain information about the timing of age-related declines and the cellular, molecular, and biochemical mechanisms employed during the aging process.

Certain species (e.g., bowhead whales) show negligible senescence over most of their long life span ***(13)***. Negligible senescence, coined by Caleb Finch ***(14)***, describes the very slow aging reported in cold-water-dwelling fish, bivalves, tortoises, and whales, many of whom are thought to live more than 100 years. Three specific criteria were proposed to test the occurrence of this phenomenon, namely (a) no predictable age-related increase in mortality rate, (b) no decrease in reproduction rate after maturity, and (c) no age-related decline in physiological capacity. Age-related naked mole-rat data (including 2- to 26-year-old animals) meet these stringent criteria. They show blunted mortality rates; maintenance of reproductive function well into the third decade of life; and only slight behavioral, biochemical, and physiological changes over a >20-year period. Proximate mechanisms facilitating these retarded

**Table 9.1** Characteristics of *r*- and *K*-selected animals

| | *r*-selected organisms | *K*-selected organisms |
|---|---|---|
| Found | Unpredictable habitats | Predictable habitats |
| Longevity | Shorter lived | Longer lived |
| Size | Smaller | Larger |
| Litter size | Larger | Smaller |
| Age at sexual maturity | Younger | Older |
| Care of offspring | Minimal | Maximal |
| Offspring survival | Lower | Higher |

Note that these are the two extremes of the *r*/*K* continuum and most animals have a preponderance of traits more in keeping with *r*- or *K*-selection but nevertheless may have some traits characteristic of either extreme. Modified from Pianka *(3)*

aging profiles may be of considerable importance in enhancing human health span well into old age.

## 9.2 Biological Features of the Naked Mole-Rat

Naked mole-rats, *Heterocephalus glaber,* are highly social bathyergid rodents naturally found in the hot, dry tropical regions of the horn of northeast Africa (Kenya, Ethiopia, and Somalia). All members of this strictly subterranean family for which longevity data are known are long-lived (Fig. 9.1), as are a few other members (e.g., porcupines) of the Hystricognath suborder to which the Bathyergidae belong. This rodent suborder includes the new world Caviomorpha (guinea pigs, tuco-tucos, and degus), the Hystricidae (porcupines), and the old world Phiomorpha (mole-rats, rock rats, and cane rats). Hystricognaths hold the record for both the largest living rodent (the Capybara, ~50 kg) and the longest-living rodent (the naked mole-rat, ~30 years) and consist of a diverse group of predominantly subterranean or semisubterranean animals ***(15)***.

Fossil evidence suggests that this rodent suborder diverged from the other main rodent suborder, the Sciurognathi, to which squirrels, beavers, mice, and rats belong, about 55 million years ago. Divergence estimates based on molecular clocks are still regarded as highly controversial ***(16)***. Earliest fossil records for the bathyergids date back to the early Miocene period [ca. 24 million years ago; ***(15, 17)***]; these fossils suggest that their ancestors have inhabited a subterranean milieu since that time and have a suite of adaptive characteristics well suited to life underground ***(18)***.

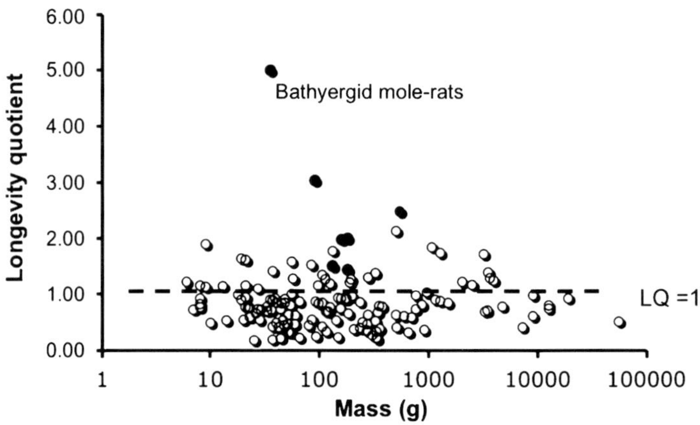


**Fig. 9.3** Longevity quotients for the rodents used in Fig. 9.1. The longevity quotient is determined using the predicted MLS based upon the allometric equation [MLS=3.34M$^{0.193}$(g)] of de Magalhães et al. (*2*) for all mammals excluding cetaceans and bats. The solid black circles represent the underground dwelling Bathyergid mole-rats

Naked mole-rats lead a strictly subterranean existence, living in large underground mazes and communally foraging for roots and tubers that are the main constituents of their herbivorous diet. Like long-lived bees, wasps, and ants, they are eusocial and live cooperatively in large colonies of up to 290 individuals [mean size, 75; ***(19)***]. In addition, they exhibit a division of labor that culminates in the presence of only a single breeding female and one to three breeding males per colony ***(11)***. Several litters of different ages remain within their natal colony throughout their lives. Young offspring receive extended care, not only from the breeding female, who nurses them for about 1 month, but also from their siblings, who collect food and carry it to the nest.

## 9.3 Age-related Changes in Mortality Rate

Rates of adult mortality do not increase with age, and deaths occur with equally low frequency in all age cohorts (Fig. 9.4) ***(20)***. As such, naked mole-rats do not show the typical age-associated acceleration in mortality risk that characterizes nearly every other species for which detailed survival data are available. Deaths occur with similar frequency in all age cohorts and do not follow the expected actuarial aging pattern of increasing mortality as animals exceed 50% of their MLS. Although we do not house animals in a barrier facility, we seldom find sick animals and, to date, have not detected measurable titers of any known rodent pathological antibodies. Furthermore, we have never observed spontaneous neoplasia in our large colony.

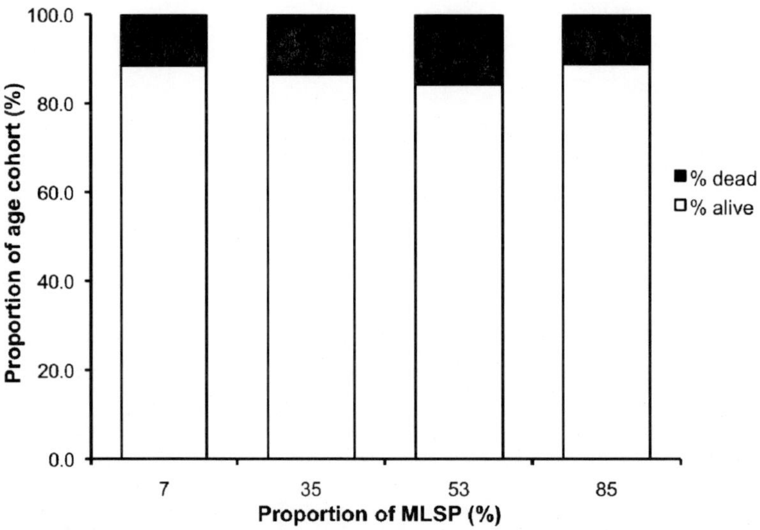


**Fig. 9.4** The proportion of individuals alive or dead in each age cohort, expressed as the proportion of maximum life span potential (MLSP)

These data confirm that naked mole-rats are extremely resilient to disease and that our record of maximum longevity may be an underestimate.

## 9.4 Reproductive Function and Age

Most evolutionary theories of aging postulate a trade-off between somatic maintenance, reproductive potential, and life expectancy. This concept forms the basis of the disposable soma theory of aging ***(4, 21)*** and suggests that animals either partition more energy into tissue maintenance or into reproductive processes. Differences in life histories and reproductive profiles among short- and long-lived species exist and are known as the *r*/*K* continuum. At the two extremes are organisms that are considered *r*- and *K*-selected (Table 9.1) ***(3)***. An *r*-selected species resides in habitats where resources are unpredictable or where predation is high and tends to exhibit fast growth rates, rapidly attain reproductive maturity, and have large litter sizes, albeit with high infant mortality (Table 9.1). Conversely, animals that reside under more stable conditions, where resource availability is more predictable, partition proportionately less energy into reproduction and more into somatic maintenance. They tend to be larger in size, breed later in life, and have smaller litters of "better quality" offspring, more likely to survive to adulthood and beyond (*K*-selected species).

Most individuals in a naked mole-rat colony never reproduce ***(11)***, and their extended longevity provides some support for the disposable soma theory of aging. Those that do breed, however, show no difference in captive life span compared with those that never breed ***(5, 22)***. Once a female becomes an established breeder and has completed her reproductive lumbar vertebrae growth surge ***(23)***, litter size (9–30 pups per litter) and reproductive output increase. Older and more established breeders produce larger litter sizes compared with young or new breeders (Table 9.2). Indeed, an age-related decline in reproductive fertility is not evident; our most successful captive-born breeding female reproduced for the last 11 years of her 23.6-year life span, reared more than 900 babies, and produced 21 pups in her last litter ***(1)***. Surprisingly, most of the older breeding females (>20 years) produce large litters, which is indicative of sustained fertility in later life ***(20)***. Further evidence

**Table 9.2** Differences in reproductive characteristics of young and old breeding females

| | Young | Old |
|---|---|---|
| Mass (g) | 37 | 45 |
| Mass increase (%) | 33 | 84 |
| Mean litter size | 9 | 16 |
| Max. litter size | 12 | 29 |
| Pup mass (g) | 1.0–2.2 | 1.0–2.4 |

Modified from Buffenstein *(20)*

of maintained fertility in old age was provided by postmortem histological data of the ovary of a wild-caught breeding female that died after 28 years in captivity. She retained many ovarian follicles at different stages of their cycle, including multiple Graafian follicles, confirming that these animals, unlike mice and humans, do not enter menopause but rather retain the capability to breed well into old age (Buffenstein, unpublished data).

This reproductive profile places naked mole-rats in an unusual position in the *r*/*K* continuum; like most rodents (e.g., mice, rats) they reproduce at a relatively young age (6 months; 2% MLS) and have large litters (up to 30 pups per litter), with comparatively high infant mortality. They, therefore, have the potential to produce an exceptionally large number of offspring over their reproductive life span. Unlike other rodents (and *r*-species in general), however, naked mole-rats exhibit *K*-selected traits as indicated by extended care of their young, the fact that they stay in their natal colony in nonreproductive states for extended periods of time, and their exceptional long life spans.

Interestingly, an 18-year demographic field study by Braude (personal communication) shows that nonbreeding individuals can be tracked for approximately 4 years whereas tagged breeding females are recaptured for at least 17 years. This finding is in sharp contrast to the <4 months most rodents, regardless of breeding status, commonly survive in the wild ***(24, 25)***. Greater life span of breeders in the wild follows a similar pattern to that observed among eusocial insects and most likely reflects the greater likelihood of extrinsic causes of mortality by either predation or accidental death in nonbreeding workers; the latter are more exposed to external dangers when leaving the nest to maintain burrow integrity or forage.

In captivity, subordinate members of the colony also exhibit extraordinary long lives as well, waiting in the sidelines should an opportunity to breed materialize. Longer life spans of breeders in the wild and similar life spans of breeders and nonbreeders in captivity are particularly surprising when the high energy demands associated with pregnancy and the extended reproductive life span are taken into account ***(26)***. Body mass may double by the end of gestation, and this increase is associated with a >1.5-fold increase in metabolic rate that increases even further to >3-fold during lactation ***(26)***. Breeding females are continuously pregnant and/or lactating throughout their long lives. Although they must partition a considerable proportion of their energy resources into reproduction, they are nevertheless able to adequately maintain both their soma and reproductive tissues far longer than do most small mammals. As such, naked mole-rat reproductive data do not support the disposable soma theory of aging.

## 9.5 Age-related changes in physiology

Long-living mole-rats maintain similar levels of physiological function for more than 20 years ***(27)***. Basal metabolic rate (BMR), gastrointestinal absorption, and enzymatic activities are maintained at similar levels, in keeping with attenuated rates of aging *(5, 27, 28)*. BMR remains unchanged for at least two-thirds of the animal's life (20 years of age; Fig. 9.5), regardless of whether it is expressed per fat-free mass or as mass-specific metabolic rate and is 30% lower than that predicted by body mass *(27)*. Reduction in oxygen consumption (and its inevitable by-product, oxidative damage) is not sufficient to account for the 5-fold difference in extended longevity compared with that predicted from body size. Given their exceptional longevity, it is not surprising that naked mole-rats have the highest mass-specific lifetime energy expenditure (LEE) of any known mammal *(27)*. This value is an underestimate of real life-time metabolic expenditure, because it does not take into account the energy expenditure for activity and is based solely upon basal, postabsorptive resting metabolic rates.

Sustained nitric oxide (NO) synthesis and nitric synthase activity may be important components of attenuated age-related changes in physiological function. NO is an important cellular signaling mechanism for maintaining normal brain, vasculature, and gastrointestinal function and has been implicated in the regulation of cellular function including protein turnover *(29)*. NO is known to exert vasculoprotective and antiatherogenic effects *(30)* and naked mole-rats appear to maintain sensitivity to NO with age (Fig. 9.6) *(31)*. Data from studies on rat arteries show substantial declines in NO-mediated dilations even in young- to middle-aged animals (14 m; 43% MLS) *(30, 32, 33)*. Conversely, sensitivity of naked mole-rat smooth muscle cells to NO does not change over a 10-year period nor does it change over a similar proportionate change in total life span *(31)*, thereby maintaining vascular and gastrointestinal functional integrity with age.

Naked mole-rats also maintain comparatively high levels of activity and mobility with age, which is achieved through efficient maintenance of bone and joints. Both bone and cartilage integrity and quality are preserved over a more than two-decade period (Fig. 9.7). No sign of articular cartilage degeneration (Pinto, Jepsen, Schaffler, and Buffenstein, unpublished data) occurs, and considerable evidence

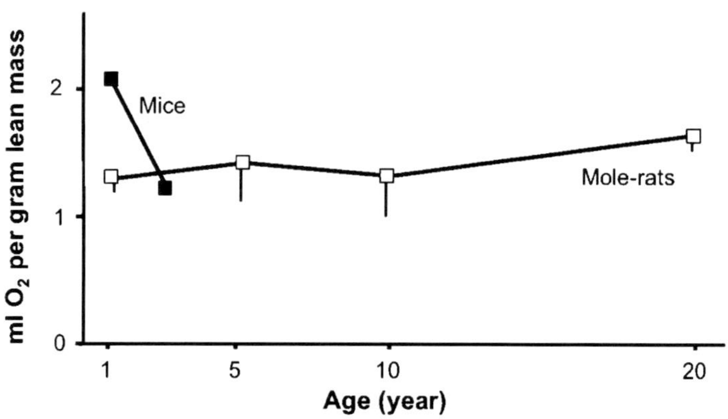


**Fig. 9.5** Age-related changes in basal metabolic rate in mice and naked mole-rats. Naked mole-rat data modified from O'Connor et al. *(27)* and unpublished data for mice

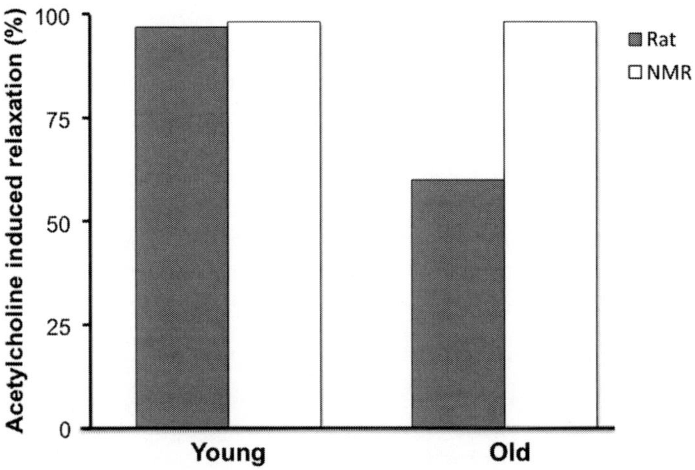


**Fig. 9.6** Unchanged sensitivity to acetylcholine in naked mole-rat blood vessels with aging. At a similar physiological age (43% of MLS), rats show a pronounced decline in blood vessel elasticity following acetylcholine exposure. Modified from Csiszar et al. *(31)*

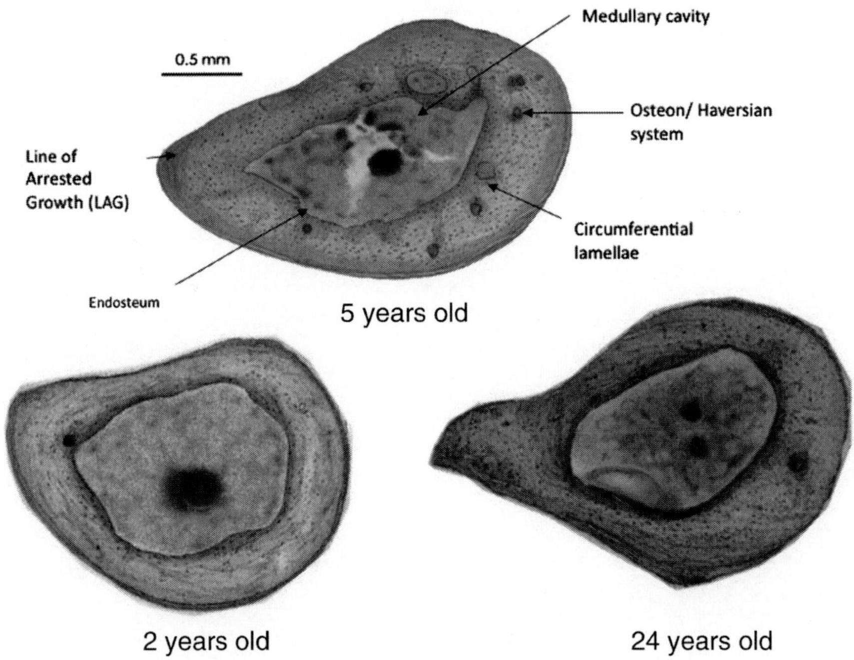


**Fig. 9.7** Cross sections through the mid shaft of the femur of young (2 years) and old (24 years) naked mole-rats. Please note that cortical bone thickness is maintained and that there are numerous signs of bone remodeling especially in the older animal (unpublished data, Y. Kramer, K. Jepsen, C. Terranova, and R. Buffenstein)

**Table 9.3** Unchanged physiological, morphological, and biochemical variables with age in naked mole-rats

| | Naked mole-rat | Mice and rats | Source |
|---|---|---|---|
| Basal metabolic rate | Unchanged | Declines | (27) |
| Nitric oxide sensitivity | Unchanged | Declines | (34) |
| Bone mineral density | Unchanged | Declines | (27) |
| Articular cartilage | Unchanged | Declines | Pinto, unpublished data |
| ROS production | Unchanged | Increases | (34) |
| Antioxidant activity | Unchanged | Increases | (35) |
| Oxidative damage | Unchanged | Increases | (36) |
| Glucose tolerance | Unchanged | Declines | (37) |
| Glycated hemoglobin | Unchanged | Declines | (28) |

exists of attenuated bone loss and efficient remodeling (Kramer, Jepsen, Pinto, Terranova, and Buffenstein, unpublished data). Maintained joint mobility coupled with resilient bone composition may contribute to the ability of old-age cohorts to move as fast as young individuals when challenged, even though, if given a choice they tend to be less active and sleep considerably longer each day than do younger individuals. Collectively, these data confirm that age-related changes in behavioral, morphological, and physiological functions of naked mole-rats are markedly attenuated (Table 9.3) and further support the premise that these small mammals show negligible senescence.

## 9.6 Age-related Changes in Biochemical and Molecular Markers

Telomeres, located at the ends of eukaryotic chromosomes, shorten with each DNA replication and cell division, and, unless continuously repaired by telomerase, telomere length controls the number of times a cell may thereby replace damaged or dying cells *(38, 39)*. The telomere shortening hypothesis postulates that, with every DNA replication, the chromosome shortens, acting as a counter for cell replication and is the cause of aging. Both humans and naked mole-rat have telomeres of similar length that are shorter than those of laboratory mice and do not correlate with their disparate longevity. Shorter telomeres, coupled with telomerase activity limited to a few actively dividing tissues [germ cells, spleen and skin tissue, Yang, Mele, Hornsby and Buffenstein unpublished data; *(40)*], may limit cell proliferation and contribute to the pronounced cancer resistance observed in naked mole-rats and humans relative to mice. Although the link between telomere length and cancer biology has considerable support, as a mechanistic theory of organismal aging, it is often contested *(41)*. Naked mole-rat data concur; clearly, proliferative potential of skin fibroblasts and its regulation by telomere length correlates more closely with body size and the total number of cells within an organism than MLS *(42)*.

The current prevailing oxidative damage theory of aging ***(43)*** postulates that slow-aging animals should produce fewer reactive oxygen species (ROS), exhibit superior antioxidant defense, and accrue less oxidative damage, allowing them longer life spans. This is not the case in naked mole-rats; production of ROS is similar to that of shorter-lived rodents ***(44, 45)***, and enzymatic antioxidant levels (e.g., catalase activity, glutathione peroxidase) are similar or lower than those of shorter-living rodents [***(35, 46)***; Yang unpublished data]. Furthermore, even from a young age, naked mole-rats exhibit high levels of oxidative damage to DNA lipids and proteins without impact upon physiological function (Fig. 9.8) [***(46)***; Perez et al., in preparation), yet they continue to live for an additional 26 years whereas young mice have fewer than 3 years of life left ***(46)***.

Naked mole-rats have markedly attenuated age-related changes in mitochondrial mass and efficiency as well as in ROS production ***(31)***, antioxidant activity ***(36)***, membrane composition ***(47)***, and lipid peroxidation ***(36)*** despite high levels of oxidative damage. In addition, although protein oxidation in particular is high, it does not accumulate with age. These adducts appear to have no impact on function (Fig. 9.9), unfolding resistance, or ubiquitination [***(48)***; Perez et al., in preparation). These data, collectively, suggest that even at the cellular level naked mole-rat functional integrity is maintained during their long lives. Efficient repair and removal of damaged macromolecules must closely match damage accrued. Tight regulation of cellular metabolism and the functional organelles involved in these processes may explain the remarkable resistance of naked mole-rat cells to a wide range of cellular insults [***(44, 49)***; Mele, Potter, and Buffenstein, unpublished data).

We do not know why naked mole-rats exhibit such high levels of oxidative damage, especially at a young age, with no impairment of function. Clearly they are

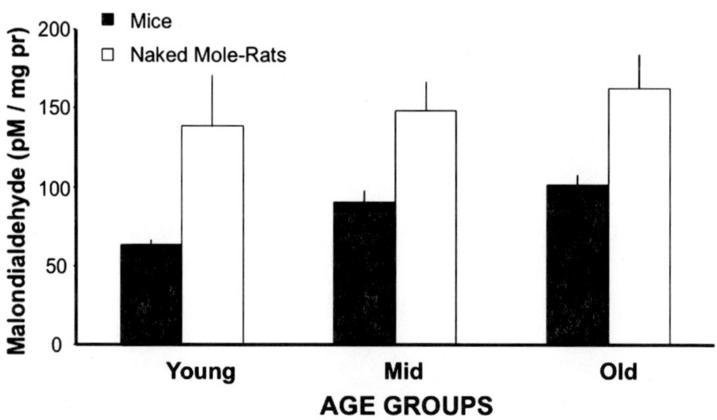


**Fig. 9.8** Age-related changes in lipid oxidation in liver tissues from naked mole-rats and mice. Note that regardless of age naked mole-rats have higher levels of oxidative damage than do mice but do not show an age-related increase in damage accrual whereas mice show an increase in accrued damage from young to middle-aged animals. Data are modified from Andziak and Buffenstein ***(36)***

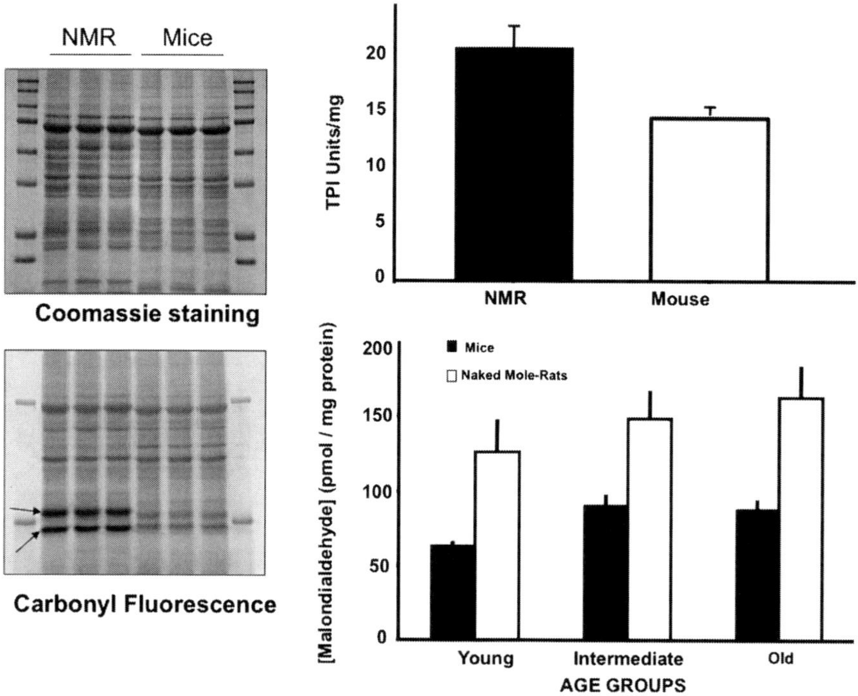


**Fig. 9.9** Naked mole-rats have considerably more protein carbonyls than do mice. Certain proteins (highlighted by *arrows*) appear to bear the brunt of this oxidative damage, one of which was identified as triosephosphate isomerase (TPI). Nevertheless, the function of this glycolytic enzyme was not impaired by the heavy presence of these adducts. Data from Andziak et al. *(35)*

extremely tolerant of this damage, showing no functional impairment, and maintain a higher steady-state threshold before damage is efficiently repaired. This higher threshold may conserve considerable amounts of energy otherwise spent on somatic repair in the face of ever-present oxidative stressors. High levels of oxidative stress with no impact on longevity and physiological function challenge the revered oxidative stress theory of aging and thus demand further investigation.

## 9.7 Conclusions

The remarkable longevity of naked mole-rats, coupled with attenuated age-related changes in morphological, physiological, biochemical, and reproductive function, suggests that these rodents possess outstanding antiaging resilience and are able to maintain somatic tissue structure and function regardless of limited telomere activity and high steady-state levels of oxidative stress. Lack of discernable age-related changes over a two-decade interval as well as pronounced cancer resistance in this mouse-sized rodent strongly suggests that naked mole-rats zealously protect their genomic integrity and rigorously maintain protein homeostasis. They thereby sustain a prolonged health span associated with slow, successful aging. Although the mechanisms enabling attenuated rates of aging remain elusive, these unusual rodents will no doubt provide novel insights into the mechanisms involved in aging, be they public or private ***(50)***, thereby facilitating their extraordinary longevity. They thus may prove to be an invaluable and useful nontraditional model for aging research and for testing the ubiquity of both ultimate and proximate theories of aging.

**Acknowledgments** Funding from the NIH/NIA is gratefully acknowledged (AG-022891). Unpublished data mentioned in the text have been collected by students Mario Pinto (CCNY), Steve Potter (UTHSCSA), and Ting Yang (CCNY), as well as by postdoctoral fellows and collaborators (Viviana Perez, James Mele, Asish Chaudhuri, and Peter Hornsby) at the Barshop Institute for Aging and Longevity Studies. Excellent animal care at the University of Cape Town, Medical School of the University of Witwatersrand, South Africa; City College of New York; and the University of Texas Health Science Center at San Antonio is gratefully acknowledged and has substantially contributed to this study.

## References

1. Buffenstein R, Jarvis JUM. The Naked Mole Rat – A New Record for the Oldest Rodent. Science's SAGE KE http://sageke.sciencemag.org/cgi/ content/full/ sageke;2002/21/pe7
2. de Magalhães JP, Costa J, Church GM. An analysis of the relationship between metabolism, developmental schedules, and longevity using phylogenetic independent contrasts. J Gerontol A Biol Sci Med Sci 2007;62:149–60.
3. Pianka ER. On r- and K-selection. Am Nat 104:592–7.
4. Ricklefs RE. Evolutionary theories of aging: confirmation of a fundamental prediction, with implications for the genetic basis and evolution of life span. Am Nat 1998;152:24–44.
5. Buffenstein R. The naked mole-rat: A new long-living model for human aging research?. J Gerontol A Biol Sci Med Sci 2005;60:1369–77.
6. Austad SN, Fischer KE. Mammalian aging, metabolism, and ecology: evidence from bats and marsupials. J Gerontol 1991;46: B47–53.
7. Heinze J, Schrempf A. Aging and reproduction in social insects – a mini review. Gerontology 2008;54:160–7.
8. Carey JR, Judge DS. Life span extension in humans is self-reinforcing: a general theory of longevity. Popul Dev Rev 2001;27:411–36.
9. Keller L, Jemielty S. Social insects as a model to study the molecular basis of ageing. Exp Gerontol 2006;41:553–6.
10. Yahav S, Buffenstein R. Huddling behaviour facilitates homeothermy in Heterocephalus glaber. Physiol Zool 1991;64:871–84.
11. Jarvis JUM. Eusociality in a mammal: cooperative breeding in naked mole-rat colonies. Science 1981;212:571–3.
12. Alexander RD, Noonan KM, Crespi BJ. The evolution of eusociality. In: Sherman PW, Jarvis JUM, Alexander RD, eds. The Biology of the Naked Mole-Rat. Princeton NJ: Princeton University Press, 1991, pp. 3–44.
13. Finch CE, Austad SN. History and prospects: symposium on organisms with slow aging. Exp Gerontol 2001;36:593–7.
14. Finch CE. Longevity, Senescence and the Genome. Chicago, IL: University of Chicago Press, 1990.

15. Bennett NC, Faulkes GG. African Mole-rats Ecology and Eusociality. Cambridge, UK: Cambridge University Press, 2000.
16. Huchon D, Madsen O, Sibbald MJ, et al. Rodent phylogeny and a timescale for the evolution of Glires: evidence from an extensive taxon sampling using three nuclear genes. Mol Biol Evol 2002;19:1053–65.
17. Lavocat R. Rodentia and Lagomorpha, In: Magio VJ, Cooke HBS, eds. Evolution of African Mammals. Cambridge, MA: Harvard University Press, 1978, pp. 69–89.
18. Buffenstein R. Ecophysiological responses to an underground habitat. In: Lacey E, Patton J, Cameron G, eds. The Biology of Subterranean Rodents. Chicago, IL: Chicago University Press, 2000, pp. 62–110.
19. Braude S. Dispersal and new colony formation in wild naked mole-rats: evidence against inbreeding as the system of mating. Behav Ecol 2000;11:7–12.
20. Buffenstein R. Negligible senescence in the longest living rodent, the naked mole-rat: insights from a successfully aging species. J Comp Physiol [B] 2008;78:439–45.
21. Kirkwood TB. Evolution of ageing. Nature 1977;24:301–4.
22. Sherman PW, Jarvis JUM. Extraordinary life spans of naked mole-rats (Heterocephalus glaber). J Zool (Lond) 2002;258:307–11.
23. O'Riain MJ, Jarvis JUM, Alexander R, Buffenstein R, Peeters C. Morphological castes in a vertebrate. Proc Natl Acad Sci U S A 2000;97:13194–7.
24. Bobeck B. Survival turnover and production of small rodents in a beech forest. Acta Theriol 1969;18:403–34.
25. Davids JHM, Jarvis JUM. Population fluctuations, reproduction and survival in the striped field mouse Rhabdomys pumilio on the Cape Flats, South Africa. J Zool (London) 1985;207:251–76.
26. Urison NT, Buffenstein R. Metabolic and body temperature changes during pregnancy and lactation in the naked mole-rat (Heterocephalus glaber). Physiol Zool 1995;68:402–20.
27. O'Connor TP, Lee A, Jarvis JUM, Buffenstein R. Prolonged longevity in naked mole-rats: Age-related changes in metabolism, body composition and gastrointestinal function. Comp Biochem Physiol A Mol Integr Physiol 2002;133:835–42.
28. Yang T, Buffenstein R. Disparate age effects on gastrointestinal enzymes in naked mole-rats. Integr Comp Biol 2002;42:1340–1.
29. Linnane AW, Kios M, Vitetta L. The essential requirement for superoxide radical and nitric oxide formation for normal physiological function and healthy aging. Mitochondrion 2007;7:1–5.
30. Csiszar A, Pacher P, Kaley G, Ungvari Z. Role of oxidative and nitrosative stress, longevity genes and poly(ADP-ribose) polymerase in cardiovascular dysfunction associated with aging. Curr Vasc Pharmacol 2005;3:285–91.
31. Csiszar A, Labinskyy N, Orosz Z, Xiangmin Z, Buffenstein R, Ungvari Z. Vascular aging in the longest-living rodent, the naked mole rat. Am J Physiol Heart Circ Physiol 2007;293:H919–27.
32. Hamilton CA, Brosnan MJ, McIntyre M, Graham D, Dominiczak AF. Superoxide excess in hypertension and aging: a common cause of endothelial dysfunction. Hypertension 2001;37:529–34.
33. Csiszar A, Ungvari Z, Edwards JG, Kaminski PM, Wolin MS, Koller A, Kaley G. Aging-induced phenotypic changes and oxidative stress impair coronary arteriolar function. Circ Res 2002;90:1159–66.
34. Csiszar A, Ahmad M, Smith KE, Labinskyy N, Gao Q, Kaley G, Edwards JG, Wolin MS, Ungvari Z. Bone morphogenetic protein-2 induces proinflammatory endothelial phenotype. Am J Pathol 2006;168:629–38.
35. Andziak B, O'Connor TP, Buffenstein R. Antioxidants do not explain the disparate longevity between mice and the longest-living rodent, the naked mole-rat. Mech Ageing Dev 2005;126:1206–12.
36. Andziak B, Buffenstein R. Disparate patterns of age-related changes in lipid peroxidation in long-lived naked mole-rats and shorter-lived mice. Aging Cell 2006;5:525–32.
37. Buffenstein R, Kang HJ, Biney A. Glucose tolerance and insulin sensitivity in an extremely long-living rodent, the naked mole-rat. FASEB J 2007;21:973.18.

38. Hayflick L. The limited in vitro lifetime of human diploid cell strains. Exp Cell Res 1965;37:614–36.
39. Von Zglinicki T. Telomeres and replicative senescence: is it only length that counts?. Cancer Lett 2001;168:111–6.
40. Harley CB, Futcher AB, Greider CW, Harley CB. Telomeres shorten during aging of human fibroblasts. Nature 1990;345:458–60.
41. Campisi J. From cells to organisms: can we learn about aging from cells in culture?. Exp Gerontol 2001;36:607–18.
42. Seluanov A, Chen Z, Hine C, Sasahara TH, Ribeiro AA, Catania KC, Presgraves DC, Gorbunova V. Telomerase activity coevolves with body mass not lifespan. Aging Cell 2007;6:45–52.
43. Harman D. Aging: a theory based on free radical and radiation chemistry. J Gerontol 1956;11:298–300.
44. Labinskyy N, Csiszar A, Orosz Z, Rivera A, Smith K, Buffenstein R, Ungvari Z. Comparison of endothelial function, O2- and H2O2 production and vascular oxidative stress resistance between the longest-living rodent, the naked mole-rat and mice. Am J Physiol 2006;291:H2698–704.
45. Lambert AJ, Boysen HM, Buckingham JA, et al. Low rates of hydrogen peroxide production by isolated heart mitochondria associate with long maximum life span in vertebrate homeotherms. Aging Cell 2007;6:607–18.
46. Andziak B, O'Connor TP, Qi W, et al. High oxidative damage levels in the longest-living rodent, the naked mole-rat. Aging Cell 2006;5:463–71.
47. Hulbert AJ, Faulks SC, Buffenstein R. Oxidation-resistant membrane phospholipids can explain longevity differences among the longest-living rodents and similarly-sized mice. J Gerontol A Biol Sci Med Sci 2006;61:1009–18.
48. Pierce AP, De Waal E, Buffenstein R, Chaudhuri A. Elevated carbonylations on specific proteins in the longest living rodent, the naked mole rat. Free Radic Biol Med 2006;41:S139.
49. Salmon AB, Amir A, Sadighi A, Buffenstein R, Miller RA. Fibroblasts from naked mole-rats are resistant to multiple forms of cell injury, but sensitive to peroxide, ultra violet light and endoplasmic reticulum stress. J Gerontol Biol Sci 2008;63A:232–41.
50. Martin GM. Keynote lecture: an update on the what, why and how questions of ageing. Exp Gerontol 2006;41:460–3.

# Chapter 10
# Life Extension in the Short-Lived Fish *Nothobranchius furzeri*

**Alessandro Cellerino**

**Abstract** Genetic and pharmacological research on aging is hampered by the life span of available vertebrate models. We recently initiated studies on *Nothobranchius furzeri,* a species with a maximum life expectancy in captivity of just 3 months, the shortest documented captive life span for a vertebrate. Further research on *N. furzeri* has demonstrated the following:

1. Short life span correlates with explosive growth and accelerated sexual maturation.
2. Short life span is correlated with the expression of age-related behavioral and histological changes.
3. Life span and expression of age-related markers can be modulated by water temperature.
4. Resveratrol, a drug characterized by its life-extending action in *Caenorhabditis elegans* and *Drosophila*, increases life span and retards expression of age-related markers.
5. Aging-related genes can be easily isolated by homology cloning.
6. Different populations or species of *Nothobranchius* show large-scale differences in captive life span.

In the last 3 years, *N. furzeri* has moved from a biological curiosity to a promising model system for drug validation. Furthermore, this species occupies a favorable position in the phylogeny of teleosts. It is close to the Japanese medaka, the puffer fishes, and the sticklebacks, and may represent a useful model for the comparative genomics of aging.

**Keywords** *Nothobranchius furzeri* • resveratrol • life span • aging

---

A. Cellerino
Fritz-Lipmann Institute for Age Research, Beutenbergstr.11, Jena, Germany.
e-mail: acellerino@fli-leibniz.de

C. Sell et al. (eds.), *Life-Span Extension,* Aging Medicine,
DOI 10.1007/978-1-60327-507-1_10,

**Abbreviations** BCT: Body core temperature; DR: Dietary restriction; GRZ: Gona Re Zhou; LF: Lipofuscin; SA-β-Gal: Senescence-associated β-galactosidase

## 10.1 Introduction

Testing the effects of experimental manipulations on life span and aging-related traits is the foundation of aging research and represents the ultimate test for aging theories. However, the life span of the available vertebrate models is a bottleneck. Mice are expensive to house, require specially built animal houses, and have a maximum life span of over 30 months for inbred mice and almost 40 months for outbred mice. Zebra fish offer many characteristics suitable for genetic manipulation and are inexpensive to maintain in large numbers compared with rodents, but their maximum life span is longer than that of mice: 58 months for an inbred strain and 66 months for an outbred strain. In other words, mice and zebra fish outlive the conventional duration of a doctoral or postdoctoral position and pose a challenge to the 3- to 5-year duration of most grants. For these reasons, longevity studies in vertebrates are attractive only to large laboratories or laboratories that are not dependent on outside funding sources.

As a consequence, only *Drosophila* or *Caenorhabditis elegans* have been adopted in systematic pharmacological studies of aging ***(1–3)***. Antioxidants, histone deacetylase inhibitors, sirtuin activators, and anticonvulsant drugs increase life span in these models ***(1–4)***. The relevance of these studies for age-related pathologic conditions is, however, questionable, given the completely different anatomical organizations of vertebrate and invertebrate bodies. Obviously, a short-lived vertebrate with a life span of a few months that shows an age-dependent physiological decline and expression of typical vertebrate age-related markers is highly desirable. A vertebrate model with an extremely rapid life cycle can be used to study drugs designed to impact vertebrate-specific genes and to assess their effects not only on longevity but also, more importantly, on age-related dysfunction of specific organ systems.

## 10.2 Teleost Fishes as a Model for Studies of Aging

The upsurge of genetic results from zebra (*Danio rerio*), medaka (*Oryzia latipes*), and, more recently, stickleback (*Gasterosteus aculeatus*) fish has demonstrated to the broad scientific community the usefulness of small bony fish as experimental and genomic models.

Teleost fish represent the most numerous group of vertebrates. As a consequence of their large numbers and their colonization of all aquatic habitats on the planet, bony fish present many extremes in vertebrate biology. For example, the smallest vertebrate *(5)*, the vertebrate with the largest sexual dimorphism (*Cryptopsaras couesii*), and the shortest-lived vertebrates are bony fish *(6, 7)*.

Fish can be housed at high-stocking density; they produce a large number of eggs that are amenable to transgenesis; transgenesis has been established in many fish species; and gene interference and large-scale mutagenesis screening have been performed in two different species of fish, medaka and zebra fish.

The first studies on aging in fish were performed by Comfort, who showed that guppies (*Poecila reticulata*) have a defined life span and that longevity can be increased by dietary restriction (DR) *(8)*. Further studies in collaboration with Woodhead demonstrated age-dependent degeneration or dysfunction of several organs *(8)*, and age-related pathological changes similar to those described in mammals were demonstrated by Liu and Walford in the annual fish *Austrolebias* *(9, 10)*. Since then, age-dependent tissue and organ degeneration has been described in a variety of fish species *(8, 11–13)*, notably in the annual fish *Nothobranchius guentheri* *(14–18)*. More recently, markers of cellular senescence, protein oxidation, and changes in heat shock proteins have been described during zebra fish aging *(13, 19)*.

A further advantage of fish is that their life span can be easily manipulated by changing water temperature *(20–22)*, and low temperature retards the expression of age-related pathologic processes *(20–22)*. Fish can also rapidly adapt to extreme changes in ambient temperature, although the influence of temperature modulation on aging in fish is, surprisingly, an almost completely neglected field.

These data demonstrate that fish are useful models for research on aging and that they share many hallmarks of aging with higher vertebrates.

Finally, those vertebrates with the shortest natural- [56 days, *Eviota sigillata*, an Australian pigmy goby *(7)*] and the shortest captive- [*N. furzeri*, 13 weeks *(6)*] life spans are teleost fish, as are some of the longest-lived vertebrates [205 years, the rockfish *Sebastes aleutianus* *(23)*]. Thus, fish are exceptional models for comparative studies of aging.

## 10.3 *N. furzeri*: An Extremely Short-Lived Vertebrate

The genus *Nothobranchius* comprises about 100 separate species, many still not described formally. These fish inhabit ephemeral pools (typically on flood plains) in eastern Africa and have adapted to the routine drying of their environment by evolving desiccation-resistant eggs that can remain dormant in the mud for one or more years *(24)*. This delay in development is accomplished by the eggs entering into diapause where oxygen consumption is depressed *(25–27)*. All of the adult fish die when the habitat dries out, and their natural life span is limited to a few or several months, making them among the shortest-lived vertebrates after the pigmy gobies of the genus *Eviota* *(7)*. Due to their short life span, annual fish were repeatedly proposed as a model system for aging research.

Our studies have focussed on the species *N. furzeri*. *N. furzeri* was originally collected in 1968 in a seasonal pan of the Gona Re Zhou (GRZ) National Park in Zimbabwe, a semi-arid area with scarce and erratic precipitation. The current laboratory strain, named GRZ after its collection point, was maintained as a pure line by dedicated hobbyists. A conservative estimate of 6 months generation time leads to a minimum of 80 captive generations. This strain must therefore be highly homozygous and comparable in genetic homogeneity to inbred strains of other laboratory species.

The median captive life span of the GRZ strain under our laboratory conditions is 9 weeks (although life span obviously depends on water chemistry, temperature, and feeding conditions and might be different in other laboratories). Interestingly, a short life span is coupled to extremely fast growth (Fig. 10.1). Under ideal culture conditions, *N. furzeri* is sexually mature and starts breeding at 3 weeks of age. *N. furzeri* GRZ is remarkably shorter-lived than the other species of the genus *Nothobranchius* for which life-history data are available, because these species show median life spans in the range of 6–12 months. The short-lived phenotype of the *N. furzeri* GRZ could stem from one of the several genetic mechanisms characteristic of closed captive populations: inbreeding depression, random drift, allele fixation, and involuntary captive selection. However, the short-lived phenotype could reflect, at least partially, an evolutionary response of the original wild population from which the founders were isolated.

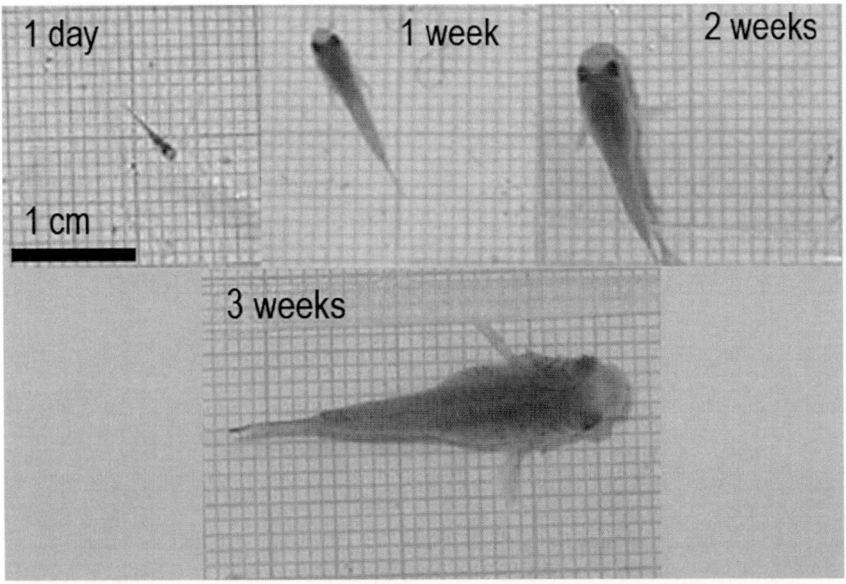


**Fig. 10.1** Growth and maturation of *N. furzeri* in captivity. The same male individual is depicted at age 1 day, 1 week, 2 weeks, and 3 weeks. At age 3 weeks, this individual was sexually mature

Classical evolutionary theories of aging predict that populations that experience low mortality due to external causes evolve retarded-onset senescence. The duration of the ephemeral pans imposes an upper limit to the natural life expectancy of different populations and species of annual fish. It is reasonable to suppose that large-scale differences in annual rainfall among different *Nothobranchius* habitats are reflected in differences in maximum natural life span and that fish inhabiting humid habitats experience longer natural life spans than fish from semi-arid habitats. The typical locality of *N. furzeri* is indeed semi-arid (about 400 mm/year of precipitation) and one of the driest areas of eastern Africa, whereas the other three species of *Nothobranchius* studied in the laboratory (*N. kunthae*, *N. rachovi*, and *N. guentheri*) originate from humid coastal habitats (about 1,600 mm/year of precipitation). These ecological differences could have led to the evolution of different aging phenotypes that are reflected in the differences in captive life span. When *Nothobranchius* species living in different habitats are compared, there appears to be a positive correlation between the length of the rainy season in the natural habitat and the life span in captivity ***(24)***. Moreover, populations of *N. furzeri* originating from more humid habitats in Mozambique show longer life spans with respect to the GRZ populations (manuscript in preparation).

The ability to raise these fish in relatively large numbers allows one to perform finely graded, age-dependent survival studies. In many organisms, death rates accelerate exponentially during midlife, but a gradual deceleration is observed later in life ***(28)***. Theoretical studies have modeled this late-life deceleration by applying a general theory of systems failure known as reliability theory ***(29)***. Late-life deceleration of death rates can be clearly observed in the laboratory strain of *N. furzeri* ***(6)***, and the best fit of the data (tested by maximum likelihood) is provided by a logistic curve (Fig. 10.2).

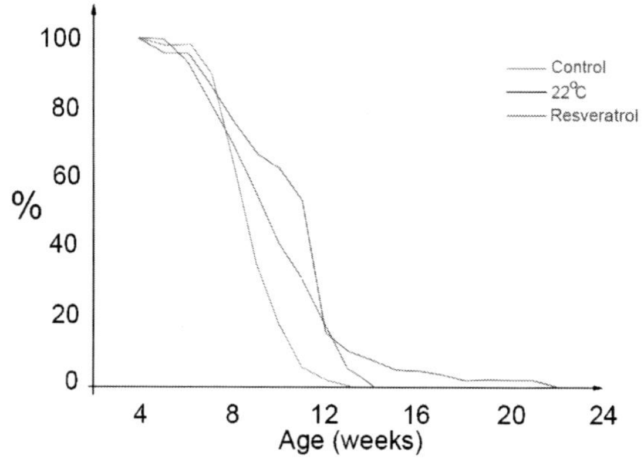


**Fig. 10.2** Life extension by temperature and resveratrol. Percentage of surviving animals is reported on the y-axis whereas age in weeks is reported on the x-axis. Experiments started at age 5 weeks when animals were sexually mature

## 10.4 Age-related Markers in *N. furzeri*

The quantification of aging rates is a key problem in biogerontology. Longevity is the most convenient end point and is the parameter commonly measured in pharmacological studies. However, longevity is also a "dirty" measure because it is often difficult to dissect the contribution of aging-related mortality from age-independent mortality due to causes such as infection, food toxicity, and unnoticed deterioration of water parameters. Therefore, the analysis of multiple end points can hardly be overemphasized. In particular, three classes of end points should be included in any analysis of aging: functional parameters, histological markers, and fertility. To validate *N. furzeri* as a model system for research on aging, it was mandatory to demonstrate that short life span is tied to an accelerated expression of age-related markers, thereby allowing one to analyze multiple end points.

Age-related reduction of locomotor efficiency is a marker for neuromuscular decay ***(30)***. We quantified spontaneous locomotor activity both in the home tank and in the open-field exploration, a standard behavioral test used for rodents that both quantifies the exploration of a new environment and shows an age-dependent decline ***(31)***. At 9 weeks of age, a decrease in both spontaneous and exploratory activity was detected ***(32)***. Learning in fish can be studied with a protocol of operative conditioning using a modification of the shuttlebox. Basically, the fish has to learn the association between the onset of a red light in one of the two compartments and a punishment. The fish can avoid punishment by moving to the other compartment within 15 s from light onset. A trial is scored as successful if the fish moves into the other compartment in response to light onset. This protocol was applied to goldfish ***(33)*** and zebra fish ***(34, 35)***, and we adapted it to *N. furzeri* ***(32)***. Young fish (5 weeks old) learned the task more rapidly than old fish (9 weeks old). This simple test reveals an age-dependent learning deficit in *N. furzeri.*

A series of histological markers of aging were detected in *N. furzeri*. One is lipofuscin (LF): LF is a conglomerate of lipids, metals, organic molecules, and biomolecules that commonly fluoresces at 360–470 nm. LF is formed within secondary lysosomes due to partially reduced oxygen species produced by mitochondria that induce lipid peroxidation and intermolecular cross-linking ***(36)***. LF accumulates with age in a variety of organs including brain, heart, and muscle in humans. LF granules have been found in every eukaryote ever examined and always accumulate within cells as the organism ages, hence its recognition as "the aging pigment." LF autofluorescence is a convenient end point because it does not require any chemical reaction to be visualized, and it can be precisely quantified by confocal microscopy ***(22, 37)***. Age-dependent accumulation of LF is observed in the liver and, to a minor extent, in the brain of *N. furzeri* ***(24)***. No accumulation of LF is observed in muscle, as reported for the zebra fish ***(13)***.

Senescence-associated β-galactosidase (SA-β-Gal) is a putative marker of cellular senescence ***(38)***. Age-dependent induction of SA-β-Gal is observed in the dermis of humans and zebra fish ***(13, 37)***. *N. furzeri* shows upregulation of SA-β-Gal at 9 weeks of age ***(24)***, which suggests that rapid induction of cellular senescence is correlated with short life span in *N. furzeri.* SA-β-Gal is a convenient marker because it does not require immunological reactions and the associated problems of cross-species antibody recognition. However, SA-β-Gal is not as easily quantified as LF. Moreover, in humans, SA-β-Gal is a lysosomal β-galactosidase whose expression is correlated with, but is not necessary for, replicative senescence ***(39)***. For this reason, SA-β-Gal should be considered an age-related marker. The demonstration of true replicative senescence in *N. furzeri* will require analysis of a larger set of markers, particularly those correlated with telomere dysfunction ***(40)***.

Finally, age-dependent neurodegeneration was demonstrated in *N. furzeri* using the specific dye Fluoro-Jade B ***(32)***. Fluoro-Jade B is a specific marker of neurofibrillary degeneration, an aging-related modification of the neuronal microtubules ***(41)***. Neurofibrillary degeneration was detected in the brain of aging salmon as well ***(42)***. It will be interesting to investigate whether other hallmarks of brain aging, such as extracellular apposition of β-amyloid or hyperphosphorylation of microtubules, are also observed in *N. furzeri.*

## 10.5 Life Extension by Temperature

Temperature variations are known to modulate aging and life-history traits in poikilotherms as different as worms, flies, and fish ***(21)***. In invertebrates, temperature modulates life span by modulating the slope of age-dependent acceleration in the death rate, which is thought to reflect the rate of age-related damage accumulation ***(43)***.

To study the effects of temperature on longevity and age-related markers in *N. furzeri*, water temperature was reduced from 25°C to 22°C after the fish reached sexual maturation (4 weeks). The treatment induced an increase of both median and maximum life span (Fig. 10.2). Life extension was linked to a reduction in the slope of the age-dependent acceleration in death rate, which suggests a reduced rate of age-related damage accumulation ***(22)***. This suggestion is further supported by the observation that reduced temperature retards the onset of age-related locomotor and learning deficits and reduces the accumulation of the age-related marker LF and of SA-β-Gal ***(22)***.

These data strongly suggest that the short life span in *N. furzeri* is tied to acceleration of the aging process. Further, these data, in combination with the early observation by Liu and Walford that reduced temperature increases longevity and retards the expression of macroscopic aging symptoms in the annual fish *Austrolebias* ***(21)***, demonstrate that reducing water temperature is a simple experimental manipulation to retard aging and age-related damage accumulation in teleosts. More recently, an ingenious transgenic mouse was created that has reduced body core temperature (BCT). In mice, a reduction of BCT of only 0.5°C is sufficient to induce detectable life extension.

Much experimental work in past decades has been devoted to the attempt to identify the molecular pathways that underlie the life-extending properties of calorie restriction. On the other hand, investigation of the molecular basis underlying the life-extending effects of temperature has been largely neglected. Only recently, two studies have examined genome-wide transcriptional response to cold adaptation in zebra fish and carp. It is of interest that cold adaptation induces upregulation of genes involved in protection from free radicals, such as SOD2, and a coordinated change in a large group of genes involved in ATP production and energy charge. This group included a number of genes that constitute complex V of the oxidative phosphorylation machinery, all of the subunits of the F1 ATP synthase complex, and components of the nonenzymatic F0 complex. This latter observation is of particular importance because upregulation of oxidative phosphorylation is also induced by resveratrol (see below), and an increase of oxidative phosphorylation could represent a common pathway between these two life-extending treatments.

## 10.6 Life Extension by Resveratrol

To date, the only molecule that consistently prolongs the life span across species and laboratories is resveratrol (3,5,4′-trihydroxyl-trans-stilbene) ***(2, 4, 44)***. This polyphenol was shown to increase the life span of yeast, *C. elegans,* and *Drosophila,* and these effects have been replicated in independent laboratories. Resveratrol is the ideal molecule with which to substantiate the suitability of *N. furzeri* as a model for drug validation. We administered resveratrol directly by mixing it with the daily food starting after the fourth week of life and continued it until death. Three different doses were administered (one dose in duplicate) plus a placebo for a total of five experimental groups and 157 fishes. Resveratrol induced a dose-dependent life extension. As in the case of reduced temperature, life extension was linked to a reduction in the slope of the age-dependent acceleration in the death rate, which suggests a reduced rate of accumulation of age-related damage. Moreover, resveratrol retarded the onset of age-dependent cognitive and locomotive deficits and prevented the expression of neurofibrillary degeneration ***(32)***. Some of these physiological changes closely resemble the changes observed in mice treated with resveratrol. Resveratrol increases the aerobic muscular performance of mice and exerts a neuroprotective action.

These results identify resveratrol as the first molecule that is able to increase the life span across animals as diverse as *C. elegans*, *Drosophila*, and fish and further highlight the importance of understanding its mechanisms of action in vertebrates. Life-long experiments with resveratrol are ongoing in mice, and it will soon be known whether resveratrol can increase the physiological life span of a vertebrate.

## 10.7 The Mechanism(s) of Action of Resveratrol

Resveratrol is a well-known molecule in the field of medical nutrition. It is a natural compound that occurs in significant amounts in red grapes and red wine; it is bioavailable when ingested and seems to be well tolerated even at extremely high doses, making it a particularly interesting candidate for the formulation of drugs.

The cardioprotective, anti-inflammatory, and antiaggregating properties of resveratrol are well documented ***(45)***. Resveratrol also shows neuroprotective activity. It protects neurons from ischemia, trauma, and excitotoxicity ***(46–50)***. Furthermore, it can induce axonal regeneration ***(51)*** and counteracts Aß toxicity by inhibition of the nuclear factor κB pathway ***(52)***. The mechanism(s) by which resveratrol induces its multiple beneficial actions are still not well defined.

An essential mediator of the effects of resveratrol in invertebrates is the NAD-dependent histone deacetylase belonging to the Sir2 (silent information regulator 2) family. Resveratrol was reported to be an activator of Sir2 in vitro. Resveratrol-induced life extension requires the presence of Sir2 in *C. elegans* and *Drosophila* ***(2)***. Overexpression of Sir2 increases the life span, and this effect is enhanced by resveratrol administration ***(44)***. Life-extending effects of DR also require Sir2 ***(53)***, and the effects of resveratrol are not observed in animals with DRs ***(2)***. It was suggested that the *sir2.1* gene is the mediator of DR effects and that resveratrol mimics the gene response induced by DR via direct activation of Sir2 ***(2)***. However, experiments in *C. elegans* indicate that resveratrol does not act upstream but rather downstream of Sir2. Moreover, Sir2 effects are totally dependent on the transcription factor Daf-16, whereas effects of resveratrol are not, an indication that they impinge on different pathways ***(44)***. Finally, even the view that DR effects are strictly dependent on Sir2 was challenged. Two independent groups have developed a protocol for DR that causes robust life extension in the worm even in the absence of Sir2 ***(54)***. Whether resveratrol effects are occluded by this new form of DR has not been tested.

Seven orthologs of the *Sir2* gene were isolated in mammals. The protein with the highest homology to Sir2 is SIRT1. SIRT1 is upregulated by DR in mammals ***(55)***. Analogous to what was observed in invertebrates, it was suggested that SIRT1 mediates the effects of DR in mammals as well.

Whether resveratrol action(s) in mammals are mediated by SIRT1 is controversial. Activation of SIRT1 can be detected only if the substrate is coupled to a fluorophore ***(56)***. In addition, the bioavailability of orally administered resveratrol is very low ***(57)***; therefore, it is impossible to achieve in vivo the concentrations needed to activate SIRT1 in vitro.

Resveratrol does, however, induce robust phenotypic effects when administered to rodents for a long term. It prevents the effects of metabolic syndrome and shifts the physiology of mice fed a high-fat diet toward that of mice fed a normal diet ***(45)***. Moreover, it induces a metabolic shift in muscle by inducing oxidative phosphorylation, mitochondrial uncoupling, a phenotypic switch from fast-twitch to slow-twitch, and an increase in aerobic endurance.

The metabolic effects of resveratrol are coupled to upregulation of the transcriptional co-factor PGC-1α ***(58)***, a key regulator of mitochondria biogenesis and energy expenditure. Many of the effects of resveratrol mimic the phenotype induced by overexpression of PCG-1α. PGC-1α is also a target of SIRT1, and upregulation and acetylation of PCG-1α in vitro are not observed in cells isolated from *sirt1*$^{-/-}$ mice. All these data suggest that the effects of resveratrol in mice are due to activation of PCG-1α via SIRT1. However, not all effects of resveratrol in mammals are dependent on SIRT1 ***(59)***.

A possibility that has not been investigated thus far is whether resveratrol induces SIRT1 at the level of gene transcription rather than at the level of enzyme activity. Surprisingly, no one has systematically investigated whether SIRT1 levels are increased in resveratrol-treated mice. An alternative possibility is that resveratrol-mediated upregulation of SIRT1 is not direct and is dependent on resveratrol-induced activation of nitric oxide synthase. Endothelial nitric oxide synthase is also induced by calorie restriction in many tissues of male mice and is responsible for many changes occurring with calorie restriction, such as mitochondrial biogenesis, increased oxygen consumption, expression of 3′-5′ guanosine monophosphate, and, importantly, SIRT1 upregulation.

## 10.8 *Nothobranchius* as a Genetic Model for Aging Studies

Additional genetic information can be obtained by whole-genome scanning techniques that identify loci controlling longevity in natural populations. One possible avenue to functional genomics of nonstandard fish models is to analyze the genotype–phenotype correlation in F2 hybrids and backcrosses of populations with markedly different phenotypes. This approach has proven highly productive in the stickleback where natural populations with markedly different morphologic characteristics can be crossed ***(63–66)***. This approach does not require sequencing of the entire genome but only that the identification of DNA polymorphic loci be used for linkage analysis and identification of genomic regions controlling the quantitative phenotypic trait under study.

Species of *Nothobranchius* from different climates show different life spans ***(24)***, and different natural populations of *N. furzeri* show large-scale differences in life span and age-related traits (manuscript in preparation). In principle, an analogous approach to the one successfully developed for the stickleback (*Gasterosteus*) can be used to identify the loci controlling longevity or aging-related phenotypic traits. In this respect, large numbers of polymorphic DNA markers for *N. furzeri* are currently being developed by the Genome Analysis Group of the Fritz-Lipmann Institute for Age Research (Jena, Germany). A first-generation linkage map is expected to be completed by 2009; this map will open the path to identification of loci controlling longevity in natural populations of *N. furzeri.*

The last necessary step in establishing a useful model for genetic studies is the ability to perform gene manipulations. Fish produce large numbers of easily accessible eggs, and transgenesis has been established in many fish species including zebra fish, medaka, and stickleback as well as in commercially relevant species such as Atlantic char, carp, channel catfish, rohu (*Labeo rohita)*, rainbow trout, tilapia, salmon, and others ***(67–77)***. In particular, the meganuclease method, a method originally developed for medaka, gave rise to efficient transgenesis in stickleback ***(78)***. Because *N. furzeri eggs* are similar in size and shape to medaka eggs, there is a realistic hope that transgenesis can be established in *N. furzeri* by applying the same technique.

## 10.9 Conclusions and Future Perspectives

In the last few years, the short-lived annual fish has demonstrated its potential as a model system for a drug validation. Because of its captive life span of only a few months, it is a good system in which to perform rapid pharmacological tests using as end point longevity as well as age-related behavioral deficits and histological modifications.

Much research so far has concentrated on the neurobiological aspects of aging. The full potential of this model system for analysis of aging-related phenotypes has yet to be realized. Age-related changes in fertility and fecundity need to be investigated systematically. The cardiovascular system has yet to be analyzed. Another crucial aspect is age-related changes in DNA, protein, and lipid oxidation. Finally, cellular senescence and telomere dysfunction need to be studied in greater detail.

The prediction is, however, that the most useful information obtained in the future will be obtained via comparative genomics. Large-scale differences in life span are observed among different subspecies and populations of *Nothobranchius* spp. In the last few years, the genes responsible for macroscopic physical differences in populations of stickleback (*Gasterosteleus* spp.) were identified by testing genotype–phenotype correlations in F2 hybrids. The same method can be applied to *Nothobranchius* to identify the genes responsible for the differences in longevity.

*Nothobranchius* occupies a favorable position in the phylogeny of teleosts. It is closely related to the Japanese medaka, whereas the puffer fish and stickleback can serve as outgroups in any analysis. In particular, large-scale analysis of expressed sequences might yield important insights into the classes of genes that have experienced positive selection or relaxation of negative selection in this short-lived vertebrate.

Finally, the possibility is strong that transgenesis can be established in *Nothobranchius* using techniques similar to those developed for medaka.

*N. furzeri* might in the future become an alternative model system for aging studies that will complement existing models. This species offers the potential of a model system in which to study drugs and to discover and characterize the genes that control the evolution of aging and senescence in natural populations.

## References

1. Kang HL, Benzer S, Min KT. 2002. Life extension in Drosophila by feeding a drug. Proc Natl Acad Sci U S A 99:838–43.
2. Wood JG, Rogina B, Lavu S, Howitz K, Helfand SL, Tatar M, Sinclair D. 2004. Sirtuin activators mimic caloric restriction and delay ageing in metazoans. Nature 430:686–9.
3. Evason K, Huang C, Yamben I, Covey DF, Kornfeld K. 2005. Anticonvulsant medications extend worm life-span. Science 307:258–62.
4. Bauer JH, Goupil S, Garber GB, Helfand SL. 2004. An accelerated assay for the identification of lifespan-extending interventions in Drosophila melanogaster. Proc Natl Acad Sci U S A 101:12980–5.

5. Kottelat M, Britz R, Hui TH, Witte KE. 2006. Paedocypris, a new genus of Southeast Asian cyprinid fish with a remarkable sexual dimorphism, comprises the world's smallest vertebrate. Proc Biol Sci 273:895–9.
6. Valdesalici S, Cellerino A. 2003. Extremely short lifespan in the annual fish Nothobranchius furzeri. Proc R Soc Lond B Biol Sci 270(Suppl 2):S189–91.
7. Depczynski M, Bellwood DR. 2005. Shortest recorded vertebrate lifespan found in a coral reef fish. Curr Biol 15:R288–9.
8. Woodhead AD. 1998. Aging, the fishy side: an appreciation of Alex Comfort's studies. Exp Gerontol 33:39–51.
9. Liu RK, Walford RL. 1970. Observations on the lifespans of several species of annual fishes and of the world's smallest fishes. Exp Gerontol 5:241–6.
10. Liu RK, Walford RL. 1972. The effect of lowered body temperature on lifespan and immune and non-immune processes. Gerontologia 18:363–88.
11. Patnaik BK, Mahapatro N, Jena BS. 1994. Ageing in fishes. Gerontology 40:113–32.
12. Gerhard GS, Kauffman EJ, Wang X, Stewart R, Moore JL, Kasales CJ, Demidenko E, Cheng KC. 2002. Life spans and senescent phenotypes in two strains of Zebrafish (Danio rerio). Exp Gerontol 37:1055–68.
13. Kishi S, Uchiyama J, Baughman AM, Goto T, Lin MC, Tsai SB. 2003. The zebrafish as a vertebrate model of functional aging and very gradual senescence. Exp Gerontol 38:777–86.
14. Markofsky J. 1976. Longitudinal and cross-sectional observations of growth and body composition with age in laboratory populations of the male annual cyprinodont fish, Nothobranchius guentheri. Exp Gerontol 11:171–7.
15. Markofsky J, Milstoc M. 1979a. Aging changes in the liver of the male annual cyprinodont fish, Nothobranchius guentheri. Exp Gerontol 14:11–20.
16. Markofsky J, Milstoc M. 1979b. Histopathological observations of the kidney during aging of the male annual fish Nothobranchius guentheri. Exp Gerontol 14:149–55.
17. Balmer RT. 1982. The effect of age on body energy content of the annual cyprinodont fish, Nothobranchius guentheri. Exp Gerontol 17:139–43.
18. Cooper EL, Zapata A, Garcia Barrutia M, Ramirez JA. 1983. Aging changes in lymphopoietic and myelopoietic organs of the annual cyprinodont fish, Nothobranchius guentheri. Exp Gerontol 18:29–38.
19. Murtha JM, Keller ET. 2003. Characterization of the heat shock response in mature zebrafish (Danio rerio). Exp Gerontol 38:683–91.
20. Liu RK, Walford RL. 1975. Mid-life temperature-transfer effects on life-span of annual fish. J Gerontol 30:129–31.
21. Yen K, Mastitis JW, Mobbs CV. 2004. Lifespan is not determined by metabolic rate: evidence from fishes and C. elegans. Exp Gerontol 39:947–9.
22. Valenzano D, Terzibasi E, Cattaneo A, Domenici L, Cellerino A. 2006a. Temperature affects longevity and age-related locomotor and cognitive decay in the short-lived fish Nothobranchius furzeri. Aging Cell 2006;5(3):275–8.
23. Cailliet GM, Andrews AH, Burton EJ, Watters DL, Kline DE, Ferry-Graham LA. 2001. Age determination and validation studies of marine fishes: do deep-dwellers live longer? Exp Gerontol 36:739–64.
24. Genade T, Benedetti M, Terzibasi E, Roncaglia P, Valenzano D, Cattaneo A, Cellerino A. 2005. Annual fishes of the genus Nothobranchius as a model system for aging research. Aging Cell 4:223–33.
25. Levels PJ, Gubbels RE, Denuce JM. 1986. Oxygen consumption during embryonic development of the annual fish Nothobranchius korthausae with special reference to diapause. Comp Biochem Physiol A 84:767–70.
26. Podrabsky JE, Hand SC. 1999. The bioenergetics of embryonic diapause in an annual killifish, Austrofundulus limnaeus. J Exp Biol 202 (Pt 19):2567–80.
27. Podrabsky JE, Hand SC. 2000. Depression of protein synthesis during diapause in embryos of the annual killifish Austrofundulus limnaeus. Physiol Biochem Zool 73:799–808.

28. Vaupel JW, Carey JR, Christensen K, Johnson TE, Yashin AI, Holm NV, Iachine IA, Kannisto V, Khazaeli AA, Liedo P, Longo VD, Zeng Y, Manton KG, Curtsinger JW. 1998. Biodemographic trajectories of longevity. Science 280:855–60.
29. Gavrilov LA, Gavrilova NS. 2004. The reliability-engineering approach to the problem of biological aging. Ann N Y Acad Sci 1019:509–12.
30. Reznick DN, Bryant MJ, Roff D, Ghalambor CK, Ghalambor DE. 2004. Effect of extrinsic mortality on the evolution of senescence in guppies. Nature 431:1095–9.
31. Furchtgott E, Wechkin S, Dees JW. 1961. Open-field exploration as a function of age. J Comp Physiol Psychol 54:386–8.
32. Valenzano DR, Terzibasi E, Genade T, Cattaneo A, Domenici L, Cellerino A. 2006b. Resveratrol prolongs lifespan and retards the onset of age-related markers in a short-lived vertebrate. Curr Biol 16:296–300.
33. Laudien H, Freyer J, Erb R, Denzer D. 1986. Influence of isolation stress and inhibited protein biosynthesis on learning and memory in goldfish. Physiol Behav 38:621–8.
34. Pradel G, Schachner M, Schmidt R. 1999. Inhibition of memory consolidation by antibodies against cell adhesion molecules after active avoidance conditioning in zebrafish. J Neurobiol 39:197–206.
35. Pradel G, Schmidt R, Schachner M. 2000. Involvement of L1.1 in memory consolidation after active avoidance conditioning in zebrafish. J Neurobiol 43:389–403.
36. Brunk UT, Jones CB, Sohal RS. 1992. A novel hypothesis of lipofuscinogenesis and cellular aging based on interactions between oxidative stress and autophagocytosis. Mutat Res 275:395–403.
37. Belichenko PV, Fedorov AA, Dahlstrom AB. 1996. Quantitative analysis of immunofluorescence and lipofuscin distribution in human cortical areas by dual-channel confocal laser scanning microscopy. J Neurosci Methods 69:155–61.
38. Dimri GP, Lee X, Basile G, Acosta M, Scott G, Roskelley C, Medrano EE, Linskens M, Rubelj I, Pereira-Smith O. 1995. A biomarker that identifies senescent human cells in culture and in aging skin in vivo. Proc Natl Acad Sci U S A 92:9363–7.
39. Lee BY, Han JA, Im JS, Morrone A, Johung K, Goodwin EC, Kleijer WJ, Dimaio D, Hwang ES. 2006. Senescence-associated beta-galactosidase is lysosomal beta-galactosidase. Aging Cell 5:187–95.
40. Herbig U, Ferreira M, Condel L, Carey D, Sedivy JM. 2006. Cellular senescence in aging primates. Science 311:1257.
41. Schmued LC, Albertson C, Slikker W, Jr. 1997. Fluoro-Jade: a novel fluorochrome for the sensitive and reliable histochemical localization of neuronal degeneration. Brain Res 751:37–46.
42. Maldonado TA, Jones RE, Norris DO. 2002. Timing of neurodegeneration and beta-amyloid (Abeta) peptide deposition in the brain of aging kokanee salmon. J Neurobiol 53:21–35.
43. Partridge L, Pletcher SD, Mair W. 2005. Dietary restriction, mortality trajectories, risk and damage. Mech Ageing Dev 126:35–41.
44. Viswanathan M, Kim SK, Berdichevsky A, Guarente L. 2005. A role for SIR-2.1 regulation of ER stress response genes in determining Celegans life span.. Dev Cell 9:605–15.
45. Baur JA, Sinclair DA. 2006. Therapeutic potential of resveratrol: the in vivo evidence. Nat Rev Drug Discov 5(6):493–506.
46. Virgili M, Contestabile A. 2000. Partial neuroprotection of in vivo excitotoxic brain damage by chronic administration of the red wine antioxidant agent, trans-resveratrol in rats. Neurosci Lett 281(2–3):123–6.
47. Kiziltepe U, Turan NN, Han U, Ulus AT, Akar F. 2004. Resveratrol, a red wine polyphenol, protects spinal cord from ischemia-reperfusion injury. J Vasc Surg 40(1):138–45.
48. Parker JA, Arango M, Abderrahmane S, Lambert E, Tourette C, Catoire H, Néri C. 2005. Resveratrol rescues mutant polyglutamine cytotoxicity in nematode and mammalian neurons. Nat Genet 37(4):349–50.
49. Raval AP, Dave KR, Pérez-Pinzón MA. 2006. Resveratrol mimics ischemic preconditioning in the brain. J Cereb Blood Flow Metab 26(9):1141–7.

50. Zamin LL, Dillenburg-Pilla P, Argenta-Comiran R, Horn AP, Simão F, Nassif M, Gerhardt D, Frozza RL, Salbego C. 2006. Protective effect of resveratrol against oxygen-glucose deprivation in organotypic hippocampal slice cultures: Involvement of PI3-K pathway. Neurobiol Dis 24(1):170–82.
51. Araki T, Sasaki Y, Milbrandt J. 2004. Increased nuclear NAD biosynthesis and SIRT1 activation prevent axonal degeneration. Science 305(5686):1010–3.
52. Marambaud P, Zhao H, Davies P. 2005. Resveratrol promotes clearance of Alzheimer's disease amyloid-beta peptides J Biol Chem 280(45):37377–82.
53. Rogina B, Helfand SL. 2004. Sir2 mediates longevity in the fly through a pathway related to calorie restriction. Proc Natl Acad Sci U S A 101(45):15998–6003.
54. Kaeberlein TL, Smith ED, Tsuchiya M, Welton KL, Thomas JH, Fields S, Kennedy BK, Kaeberlein M. 2006. Life span extension in Caenorhabditis elegans by complete removal of food. Aging Cell 5(6):487–94.
55. Picard F, Kurtev M, Chung N, Topark-Ngarm A, Senawong T, Machado De Oliveira R, Leid M, McBurney MW, Guarente L. 2004. Sirt1 promotes fat mobilization in white adipocytes by repressing PPAR-gamma. Nature 429(6993):771–6.
56. Borra MT, Smith BC, Denu JM. 2005. Mechanism of human SIRT1 activation by resveratrol. J Biol Chem 280(17):17187–95.
57. Wenzel E, Somoza V. 2005. Metabolism and bioavailability of trans-resveratrol. Mol Nutr Food Res 49(5):472–81.
58. Lagouge M, Argmann C, Gerhart-Hines Z, Meziane H, Lerin C. 2006. Resveratrol improves mitochondrial function and protects against metabolic disease by activating SIRT1 and PGC-1alpha. Cell 127(6):1109–22.
59. Zhang J. 2006. Resveratrol inhibits insulin responses in a SirT1-independent pathway. Biochem J 397(3):519–27.
60. Muller F. 2005. Comparative aspects of alternative laboratory fish models. Zebrafish 2:47–54.
61. Miya M, Takeshima H, Endo H, Ishiguro NB, Inoue JG, Mukai T, Satoh TP, Yamaguchi M, Kawaguchi A, Mabuchi K, Shirai SM, Nishida M. 2003. Major patterns of higher teleostean phylogenies: a new perspective based on 100 complete mitochondrial DNA sequences. Mol Phylogenet Evol 26:121–138.
62. Kim IC, Lee JS. 2004. The complete mitochondrial genome of the rockfish Sebastes schlegeli (Scorpaeniformes, Scorpaenidae). Mol Cells 17:322–8.
63. Peichel CL, Nereng KS, Ohgi KA, Cole BL, Colosimo PF, Buerkle CA, Schluter D, Kingsley DM. 2001. The genetic architecture of divergence between threespine stickleback species. Nature 414:901–5.
64. Shapiro MD, Marks ME, Peichel CL, Blackman BK, Nereng KS, Jonsson B, Schluter D, Kingsley DM. 2004. Genetic and developmental basis of evolutionary pelvic reduction in threespine sticklebacks. Nature 428:717–23.
65. Colosimo PF, Hosemann KE, Balabhadra S, Villarreal G, Jr., Dickson M, Grimwood J, Schmutz J, Myers RM, Schluter D, Kingsley DM. 2005. Widespread parallel evolution in sticklebacks by repeated fixation of Ectodysplasin alleles. Science 307:1928–33.
66. Kimmel CB, Ullmann B, Walker C, Wilson C, Currey M, Phillips PC, Bell MA, Postlethwait JH, Cresko WA. 2005. Evolution and development of facial bone morphology in threespine sticklebacks. Proc Natl Acad Sci U S A 102:5791–96.
67. Dunham RA, Ramboux AC, Duncan PL, Hayat M, Chen TT, Lin CM, Kight K, Gonzalez-Villasenor I, Powers DA. 1992. Transfer, expression, and inheritance of salmonid growth hormone genes in channel catfish, Ictalurus punctatus, and effects on performance traits. Mol Mar Biol Biotechnol 1:380–9.
68. Hew CL, Davies PL, Fletcher G. 1992. Antifreeze protein gene transfer in Atlantic salmon. Mol Mar Biol Biotechnol 1:309–17.
69. Male R, Lorens JB, Nerland AH, Slinde E. 1993. Biotechnology in aquaculture, with special reference to transgenic salmon. Biotechnol Genet Eng Rev 11:31–56.

70. Alam MS, Lavender FL, Iyengar A, Rahman MA, Ayad HH, Lathe R, Morley SD, Maclean N. 1996. Comparison of the activity of carp and rat beta-actin gene regulatory sequences in tilapia and rainbow trout embryos. Mol Reprod Dev 45:117–22.
71. Rahman MA, Mak R, Ayad H, Smith A, Maclean N. 1998. Expression of a novel piscine growth hormone gene results in growth enhancement in transgenic tilapia (Oreochromis niloticus). Transgenic Res 7:357–69.
72. Krasnov A, Agren JJ, Pitaknen TI, Molsa H. 1999. Transfer of growth hormone (GH) transgenes into Arctic charr. (Salvelinus alpinus L.) II. Nutrient partitioning in rapidly growing fish. Genet Anal 15:99–105.
73. Nam YK, Cho YS, Kim DS. 2000. Isogenic transgenic homozygous fish induced by artificial parthenogenesis. Transgenic Res 9:463–9.
74. Nam YK, Noh JK, Cho YS, Cho HJ, Cho KN, Kim CG, Kim DS. 2001. Dramatically accelerated growth and extraordinary gigantism of transgenic mud loach Misgurnus mizolepis. Transgenic Res 10:353–62.
75. Zbikowska HM. 2003. Fish can be first – advances in fish transgenesis for commercial applications. Transgenic Res 12:379–89.
76. Morita T, Yoshizaki G, Kobayashi M, Watabe S, Takeuchi T. 2004. Fish eggs as bioreactors: the production of bioactive luteinizing hormone in transgenic trout embryos. Transgenic Res 13:551–7.
77. Wu B, Sun YH, Wang YP, Wang YW, Zhu ZY. 2004. Sequences of transgene insertion sites in transgenic F4 common carp. Transgenic Res 13:95–6.
78. Hosemann KE, Colosimo PF, Summers AT, Kingsley DM. 2004. A simple and efficient microinjection protocol for making transgenic sticklebacks. Behaviour 141:1345–56.

# Part VI
# Aging in Humans

# Chapter 11
# Aging and Longevity in Animal Models and Humans

**Miriam Capri, Stefano Salvioli, Elisa Cevenini, Laura Celani, Federica Sevini, Elena Bellavista, Catia Lanzarini, Stella Lukas, Paolo Tieri, Francesco Lescai, Daniela Monti, and Claudio Franceschi**

**Abstract** How many animal models are adequate to study human aging? Aging is an adaptive process performed by an integrated panel of evolutionarily selected mechanisms aimed at maintaining soma integrity. The possibility of extrapolating results from animal models to human beings has to be addressed in an ecological context. Model systems fit basic requirements of scientific research, and experimental animals show a series of advantages for the study of aging and longevity in humans. However, animal models have intrinsic constraints because they are artificial: Humans are not inbred and live in different conditions from both an environmental and a socio-anthropological-cultural point of view. Even if research on aging and longevity has been performed primarily in model systems such as yeast, worms, and flies, results obtained in humans are not only of basic importance but are also largely unexpected, probably because of the peculiar characteristics of humans (protected environment, culture, economic conditions, stochasticity). In some cases, studies in animal models or humans have led to analogous results, largely because basic mechanisms involved in aging have been conserved throughout evolution. In other cases, results are different or even opposite, as is described in this chapter. Animal models are often not sufficiently adequate for the study of human longevity, but their usefulness in achieving knowledge at different levels (molecular, cellular, physiological, behavioral) is unquestionable. Thus, it seems that the concomitant and integrated use of *ad hoc* models, also comparing different species, together with new *in silico* and high throughput strategies, will be the general framework within which studies on human aging and longevity should be performed to accelerate the identification of new determinants of healthy aging and longevity.

M. Capri, S. Salvioli, E. Cevenini, L. Celani, F. Sevini, E. Bellavista,
C. Lanzarini, S. Lukas, P. Tieri, F. Lescai, and C. Franceschi (✉)
Department of Experimental Pathology, University of Bologna, Via S. Giacomo 12, 40126, Bologna, Italy
C.I.G.-Interdepartmental Centre "L. Galvani," University of Bologna, Via Selmi 3, 40126, Bologna, Italy
e-mail: claudio.franceschi@unibo.it

D. Monti
Department of Experimental Pathology and Oncology, University of Florence, Florence, Italy

C. Sell et al. (eds.), *Life-Span Extension*, Aging Medicine,
DOI 10.1007/978-1-60327-507-1_11,

**Keywords** Aging • longevity • animal models • p66shc • PON1 • nuclear factor-κB • TP53 • SIRT1 • insulin-like growth factor I • caloric restriction

**Abbreviations** CR: Caloric restriction; FOXO1A: Forkhead box 01A; IGF-I: Insulin-like growth factor I; IGF-IR: Insulin-like growth factor I receptor; NF-κB: Nuclear factor-κB; PI3KCB: Phosphoinositide 3-kinase; PON1: Paraoxonase 1; VNTR: Variable number tandem repeat

## 11.1 Human Aging and Longevity Within an Evolutionary Perspective

Human longevity is determined by the interaction of genetic, epigenetic, and environmental components with stochastic factors. Aging should be considered a dynamic process leading to continuous adaptation of the body to the life-long exposure to harmful stressors, as conceptualized in the remodeling theory of aging *(1, 2)*. These stressors include damaging agents, produced by the organism as a consequence of inescapable physiological metabolic processes (e.g., reactive oxygen species, from oxidative metabolism), as well as those derived from exposure to a variety of physical (e.g., ultraviolet rays from sun exposure) and biological (viruses, bacteria, parasites) agents. Collectively, they represent the *environment* into which the body is plunged. The body has to counteract and neutralize the negative effects of such stressors with a panel of antistressor mechanisms. Stressors acting at different levels include the following:

- *Molecular stressors*: they induce heat shock protein and other chaperone protein production, increased protein and organelle turnover, antioxidant and detoxifying systems, and DNA repair mechanisms.
- *Cellular stressors*: they induce apoptosis and autophagic cell death (or cell senescence), phagocytosis and scavenging of damaged cells, and replacement of dead cells by progenitors derived from stem cells (cell and tissue renewal).
- *Systemic stressors:* they stimulate immune and inflammatory responses, stress responses, and neuroendocrine responses.
- *Organismal stressors*: they alter behavioral responses designed to minimize danger and damage.

All these integrated responses, which also depend on stressor types and exposure time, contribute to survival. It can be predicted that the global rate of aging and the maximum life span (final longevity) attained by a species is equal to (or greater than) the sum of all these mechanisms (adaptation or remodeling capacity for each species). During evolution, a positive selection process occurred to maximize the overall efficiency of these defense mechanisms because they were critical to maintain a healthy status and to maximize reproductive capacity and fitness. This is the main reason why, from an evolutionary perspective, we may assume that the fundamental biological mechanisms playing a major role in the aging process are highly conserved throughout evolution, and that, accordingly, extrapolation from model systems to humans is reasonable. Comparative data on single genes or gene families throughout evolution fit with this assumption. It is also clear that, despite such a conservative scenario, major changes occurred in evolution, particularly regarding biological regulatory processes and integration between and among pathways, and that major differences among species also emerged during evolution. This consideration is particularly important for *Homo sapiens* and his biologic characteristics, including aging. Moreover, from an ecological systemic perspective of the different life spans of various species, it is possible to assume that, owing to the extremely complex relationship and interactions among different species in a defined environment and the reciprocal constraints in terms of predator/prey, their life spans should fit a general, ecological equilibrium. In other words, we can speculate that the unexpected *plasticity and malleability* of the aging process and longevity that are emerging in biogerontologic studies have a strong evolutionary basis, being a prerequisite for adaptation to ecological changes that require a plastic, malleable life span of all the species present in a specific environment, in order to attain a general ecological equilibrium among species.

Therefore, we may predict that the variable longevity of individuals within a species can be explained by assuming a different individual adaptation and remodeling capacity. This capacity is based on subtle differences among individuals regarding the efficiency of the above-mentioned set of defense mechanisms, evolutionarily selected for a certain level of efficiency in each species as a whole. Thus, aging is an adaptive process (remodeling) modulated by an integrated panel of evolutionarily selected mechanisms. The possibility of extrapolating results from animal models to human beings has to be addressed in an ecological context, starting from animal models as a basis for elucidating the aging process in humans.

## 11.2 Advantages and Successes of Model Systems: The Crucial Importance of the Reductionist Approach

The essential role of the ecological niche or habitat is evident if we take into account some domesticated animals. They can attain longer or shorter lives than if they were living in their wild habitat. The reasons may be new life style, change of diet, disease, or absence of predators. The maximum life span of a given animal is determined by factors such as species-specific genes and environmental and stochastic factors, in a way similar to humans but the importance of the different ingredients probably differs quantitatively and qualitatively.

A variety of model systems have been developed to assess the role played by the above-mentioned antistressor mechanisms in the aging process. DNA repair mechanisms ***(3–5)***, telomere length, telomerase activity, and all of the previously mentioned processes have been studied in different animal models ***(6–8)***. Comparative studies of stress resistance in primary cultures ***(9, 10)*** showed that cells from long-lived species are indeed better protected by somatic maintenance and repair mechanisms.

Ultimately, birds may be considered the more suitable models of longevity than the short-lived laboratory rodents. Studies in birds may reveal routes for therapeutic intervention in diseases of human aging ***(11)***.

Animal models have been used in all fields of biology and genetics of aging with remarkable success. This approach is reductionist by definition and the basic assumption is that the simpler the organism, the more successful will be the investigation on the fundamental "cause" of aging and longevity. Model systems fit basic requirements of scientific research. Indeed, experimental animals have the following advantages for the study of aging and longevity: (1) they are inexpensive, can be easily handled, and reproduce quickly; (2) they are well-characterized genetically (usually pure inbreed strains); (3) their environment is well controlled (feasible to change environmental conditions) and constant. These advantages assure the possibility to replicate the results in different laboratories (reproducibility), another basic requirement of scientific research.

## 11.3 Disadvantages and Intrinsic Constraints of Model Systems

Animal models have intrinsic constraints because they are artificial. Humans are not inbred and live in remarkably different conditions from both environmental (climate, food, and water availability; exposure to pathogens) and socio-anthropological-cultural (economic conditions, availability of social and medical care) points of view. In particular, the disadvantages of animal models are as follows:

1. Life span is frequently measured in knockout animals created in the laboratory under controlled conditions. It is, therefore, necessary to consider the meaning of an increase or a decrease in the life span of such animal models because it is difficult to predict the effective role of these mutations and how long these animals could survive in the wild and adapt themselves to frequently changing environmental conditions (such as temperature, food availability, predators). Knockout animals are far from an evolutionary setting. Moreover, we should be careful in transferring the results to humans. We can assume that our genetic variants have been selected by evolution to enable us to survive in conditions completely different from those in which we currently live.
2. The entire aging process of animal models such as *Drosophila melanogaster* and *Caenorhabditis elegans* (invertebrates) differs from that of humans because the former are composed mainly of postmitotic cells that are unable to proliferate (postmitotic animals). In contrast, higher vertebrates and humans are composed of both postmitotic and proliferating cells, with stem cells able to generate new cells that replace the damaged and dead ones. Although we have learned a great

deal about developmental biology from worms, flies, and mice, detailed information on the pathophysiology of aging and on the variations among genetically heterogeneous wild-type populations, particularly worms and flies, is scarce. In contrast, the literature on these and all other aspects of human biology, including remarkable progress in human genetics, is extensive. Moreover, physicians have provided detailed descriptions of late-in-life disabilities and diseases, including cancer in human populations. *D. melanogaster* and *C. elegans* do not seem to undergo similar pathologic processes ***(12)***.

3. Additional, unique DNA sequences have evolved in *H. sapiens*, including rapidly evolving and functionally significant intronic sequences that distinguish us from our nearest relative, the common chimpanzee (*Pan troglodytes*), whose life span is approximately half that of humans ***(13, 14)***.
4. A major problem with studies of the immune system is the fact that animal models live in pathogen-free conditions in which it is not possible to evaluate parameters such as the role of climate, food intake, water availability, infections onset, and intestinal flora. Moreover, in *D. melanogaster* and *C. elegans,* the immune system is composed only of innate immunity, whereas in the mouse, adaptive immunity is also present, but the life span is short and not comparable to the human life span.
5. Studies on the effect of the large number of mitochondrial DNA genetic variants on aging and longevity are appropriately performed only in humans because of the specific evolutionary history of *H. sapiens*. This example illustrates the important, peculiar interconnection between the evolutionary history of a species and the determinants of its longevity.
6. Genetic studies on humans, especially centenarians, performed in different European countries were often not reproducible. The reasons are complex and are due, at least in part, to the fact that the centenarian phenotype is highly heterogeneous ***(15)***. Such differences are of great general interest and may account for many problems of reproducibility of the genetic studies on human longevity ***(16)***. Indeed, we believe that genetic studies should not always and necessarily be reproducible in different populations because the centenarian phenotype and, in general, human aging are the results of a complex relationship between genetics and the environment (postreproductive or unusual genetics of centenarians). These peculiar interactions, unique for each individual, contribute to the substantial heterogeneity of the aging process. Some of the characteristics are shared by many individuals or groups, whereas others are "private" ones – mechanisms that are present only in particular subsets of individuals or even in single individuals ***(17–19)***. *H. sapiens* shows a higher level of complexity and heterogeneity than do other animal models, even if this level of complexity seems more correlated with the number of DNA spacer sequences than with the number of genes. The number of cellular identities also can give a measure of human complexity when compared with those of other species. It has been calculated that *C. elegans*, which is composed of about 18,000 genes and 1,179 somatic cells (in males) or 1,090 somatic cells (in females) precisely mapped, have $10^3$ cellular identities, taking into account their specific ontogeny and their

positional identity. *H. sapiens*, which is composed of about 25,000 genes and $10^{14}$ somatic cells, most of which are precisely localized with a specific organized architecture, has about $10^{12}$ cellular identities.

In conclusion, we can argue that the approach that exploits model systems must be enriched and integrated. Studies on humans are the best way to study human aging and longevity because, despite the effort required to perform studies on human beings, they cannot be replaced by studies on model systems because of the peculiarities of *H. sapiens* from a biological and a cultural-anthropological point of view ***(12, 20)***.

## 11.4 Studies on Human Aging and Longevity

Even if research on aging and longevity has been dominated by studies performed in model systems such as yeast, worms, and flies, the results obtained in humans are not only of primary importance but are largely unexpected, probably because of the peculiar biological characteristics of humans. The long 9-month in utero developmental period is several times longer than the entire life span of some animal models. Moreover, the placental type of reproduction typical of mammals implies a complex relationship between the mother and the fetus. A similar situation (although much shorter) is found in mice. The amount of information that the mother can deliver to and exchange with the fetus, as a consequence of her nutritional status, antigenic exposure, and emotional stress, among others, does not have an equivalent in most experimental models. A variety of data indicate that nutritional problems of the fetus, such as low birth weight, can have long-term effects on the onset of diabetes or cardiovascular disease ***(21, 22)***. It is not known whether these situations have long-term effects on survival and on human aging and longevity. Thus, these types of studies are urgently needed. Similar considerations apply to the possible effects on the offspring of infectious diseases occurring during specific periods (windows) of pregnancy. A variety of data in mice indicate that the inflammatory cytokines produced by the mother can cross the placenta and have profound behavioral effects on the developing brain, which appears to be sensitive to cytokines ***(23)***.

It has recently been argued that the rules of the aging process must be traced back to the fetal developmental events that established constraints that represent major determinants of the process ***(24)***, thus extending the antagonistic pleiotropy theory of aging ***(25)***. We argued that antagonist pleiotropy is important and more common than previously thought ***(16)***. The entire aging process can be considered an *antagonistic maladaptive process*, mainly because of an evolutionary discrepancy between our body, molded by evolution during millions of years, and our present environment, drastically changed in the last centuries. In any case, the length of human development in utero as well as until the age of reproduction and the importance of cultural training and education in this developmental process suggest that specific mechanisms probably emerged in humans that can have a pleiotropic effect on the rate of aging and an impact on human longevity ***(26)***.

## 11.5 Similar Results on Longevity Among Species

Because human aging is the product of interactions among factors in which genetics plays only a part, we wish to stress that it is not always possible to extrapolate results to humans from animal models in which most of these variables have been eliminated or controlled, e.g., cultures of mutated *C. elegans* or knockout/transgenic mice. In few cases, studies on the genetics of longevity led to similar results in both animal models and humans.

### *11.5.1 SIRT3*

The human *sirtuin 3* gene encodes a putative mitochondrial NAD-dependent deacetylase (SIRT3) that belongs to an evolutionarily conserved family of proteins named sirtuins. Studies in model organisms demonstrated the role of the *Sir2* gene in life span extension ***(27, 28)***. Our study suggests that polymorphism of the *SIRT3* gene (G477T transversion) is associated in humans with a gender-specific effect on longevity (in elderly men, the TT genotype increases survival, whereas the GT genotype decreases it) ***(29)***. Because the G477T transversion does not change the amino acid in the conserved sirtuin domain, the observed association could be due to a linkage disequilibrium with either a functional variant of the *SIRT3* gene itself or other neighboring genes. In fact, *SIRT3* lies in a chromosomal region (11p15.5) where four genes potentially associated with longevity are located (*HRAS1*, insulin-like growth factor 2, proinsulin, and tyrosine hydroxylase) ***(29)***. More recently, a variable number tandem repeat (VNTR) polymorphism (72-bp repeat core) in intron 5 of the human *SIRT3* gene has been described ***(30)***. This VNTR region seems to have allele-specific enhancer activity. Studies on the frequency of this polymorphism indicated that the allele lacking enhancer activity is virtually absent in men older than 90 years ***(30)***. Thus, underexpression of this human *sirtuin* gene seems to be detrimental for longevity suggesting that sirtuin gene family members are involved in longevity in both model systems and humans.

### *11.5.2 Insulin and Insulin-Like Growth Factor-I Signaling Pathway*

Genes that encode components of this pathway are strong candidates for longevity in humans as well as in animal models. In yeast, worms, and flies, the partially conserved glucose or insulin/insulin-like growth factor I (IGF-I)-like pathways downregulate antioxidant enzymes and heat shock proteins, reduce the accumulation of glycogen or fat, and control growth and mortality. Mutations that reduce the activity of these pathways appear to extend longevity by simulating caloric restriction (CR) or more severe forms of starvation. In yeast and worms, the induction of stress-resistance genes is required for longevity extension. In mice, IGF-I activates signal transduction pathways analogous to the longevity regulatory pathways in lower eukaryotes and increases mortality ***(31)***. In addition, in animal models such as the mouse, the downregulation of the IGF-I pathway is associated with an extension of life span ***(32–34)***, whereas high levels of IGF-I are associated with a shortened life span ***(34)***.

We investigated polymorphisms in humans at the IGF-I receptor (*IGF-IR*), phosphoinositide 3-kinase (*PI3KCB*), insulin receptor substrate-1 (*IRS-1*), and forkhead box 01A (*FOXO1A*) genes as well as their possible effects on IGF-I plasma levels ***(35, 36)***. These genes represent key molecules of the insulin/IGF-I pathway, and their sequential activation determines a cascade activation signal. Our study was performed with 496 healthy Caucasian subjects subcategorized into two groups (85+ and younger than 85 years). The study results indicated that free IGF-I plasma levels displayed an age-related decrease and that these levels were affected by the polymorphisms at the *IGF-IR* and *PI3KCB* genes. The polymorphisms considered in the study were a G to A transition at nucleotide 3,174 in exon 16 of the *IGF-IR* and a T to C transition located 359 bp upstream from the starting codon of *PI3KCB*. Again, the presence of at least one A allele at the *IGF-IR* locus was shown to result in low levels of free-plasma IGF and to be more highly represented among long-lived individuals. The same study also reported that different combinations of *IGF-IR* and *PI3KCB* alleles affect free-plasma IGF-I levels and longevity.

Using a different approach, van Heemst et al. ***(37)*** carried out a longitudinal study of two cohorts of individuals who were at least 85-years old. They assessed components of the insulin/IGF-I pathway in these cohorts. The study indicated that genetic variation causing reduced insulin/IGF-I activation is beneficial for survival in old age, but only for women. When the polymorphisms of IGF-IR and PI3KCB were considered together, another interesting result emerged. The proportion of IGF-IR/PI3KCBAβ/Tβ carriers was significantly increased among long-lived individuals.

### *11.5.3 TP53*

*TP53* is a master gene involved in several molecular pathways such as apoptosis, cell senescence, DNA repair, and cell cycle arrest. *TP53* has long been considered a longevity-assurance gene in the sense that it acts on longevity by preventing tumors, since p53-deficient mice have a shorter life span than their normal counterparts because of rapid development of tumors ***(38)***. Nevertheless, in the case of p53-competent animals, the situation is likely more complicated and controversial. It has been observed that, in mice, the gain of function of p53 led to increased tumor suppression but also decreased longevity, probably because of a deleterious effect on stem cell proliferative capability ***(39)***. Mice expressing a deleted form of p53 that confers a gain of function display protection from cancer onset; they also express early onset of phenotypes associated with aging, which include reduced longevity, osteoporosis, generalized organ atrophy, and diminished stress tolerance. A second line of transgenic mice containing a temperature-sensitive mutant allele of p53 also exhibits similar features ***(39)***. It was thus hypothesised that p53 activity against cancer occurred at the expense of longevity. This tenet has been challenged by the finding that a peculiar TP53 transgenic mouse has increased tumor suppression and ages normally ***(40)***. This super-p53 mouse has supernumerary copies of the *TP53* gene in the form of large genomic transgenes. These supernumerary copies of *TP53* are surrounded by regulatory sequences identical to those at the endogenous *TP53* locus. The *TP53* gene is thus under normal regulatory control, which avoids the abnormal overexpression to which the deleterious side effects (premature aging) are likely to be ascribed. Also in humans, the *TP53* gene can be considered a longevity assurance gene in the sense that it effectively avoids tumorigenesis. Indeed, it is found to be mutated in half of human cancers ***(41)***, and it is completely lacking in a rare inherited genetic disease featuring early cancer onset (Li-Fraumeni syndrome). It is not yet clear whether common variants of this gene are associated with longevity or accelerated aging in humans. A common functional polymorphism at codon 72 in the *TP53* gene has been widely studied. This polymorphism, determining an arginine (R) to proline (P) amino acid substitution in the p53 protein, modulates the susceptibility to apoptosis and cell senescence in old people in ex vivo experiments. Our group and others observed that cells from individuals homozygotic for the R allele (RR) undergo apoptosis to a greater extent than cells obtained from P allele carriers (P+) ***(42, 43)***. Furthermore, we and others observed that the P53P72 isoform is more able than the P53R72 isoform to promote stress-induced cell senescence in dermal fibroblasts obtained from elderly people and centenarians but not from young people ***(44, 45)***. Given these consistent biological differences, as well as the number of reports indicating different risk of many types of cancers for the two p53 isoforms, we hypothesized an association of the codon 72 polymorphism of *TP53* gene with longevity. Early studies from our group indicated that this polymorphism was not differently distributed among age classes, including centenarians, in the Italian population ***(46)***. Nevertheless, a more recent study reported a meta-analysis indicating that subjects carrying the *TP53* codon 72 proline allele have a survival advantage despite a higher risk of cancer in long-lived people ***(47)***. These results have been partially confirmed in another study in the Danish population in which the authors suggest that the increased longevity of *TP53* codon 72 proline allele carriers may be due to increased survival after a diagnosis of cancer or other life-threatening diseases ***(48)***. It is possible that the genetic frequencies found in Italians are the result of the interaction between the *TP53* gene and other gene variants peculiar to Italians but not to other populations.

### *11.5.4 Nuclear Factor-κB System*

The nuclear factor-κB (NF-κB) system is a conserved signaling pathway that plays a key role in regulating the immune response in mammals. NF-κB and IκB homologs with immune-related functions have been identified in evolutionarily distant organisms. In *Drosophila melanogaster* and *Anopheles gambiae*, NF-κB homologs (Dorsal, Dif, Relish, and REL2 respectively) are responsible for regulating humoral immunity and expression of immune effectors ***(49, 50, 51)****. In Carcinoscorpius rotundicauda* (limulus, or horseshoe crab) a primitive and functional NF-κB pathway can regulate the expression of immune-related genes *in vivo* (inducible nitric oxide synthase -iNOS- and *Carcinoscorpius rotundicauda* Factor C, the LPS-activated enzyme that triggers the coagulation cascade in immune defense) ***(52)***. Unexpectedly, in *Caenorhabditis elegans*, the NF-κB protein is absent, and similar functional homologs (Cactus, Toll, Traf) seem to be not involved in innate immune response ***(53)***.

The role of NF-κB signaling in the aging process can be studied in different aging models in terms of the interactions of the NF-κB system, and related inflammatory processes, with gerontogenes and age-related signaling networks. In this perspective, recent studies indicate that yeast and *Caenorhabditis elegans* models exhibit common features with mammalian aging ***(54)***. It has been demonstrated that Sir2 (mammalian sirtuins homolog) is a key regulator of aging in budding yeast, a popular model in aging research. Even if there is no evidence that mammalian aging is sirtuin-dependent ***(55, 56)***, sirtuins have proven to be important proteins in cellular metabolism and then linked to several age-related disease and aging.

In *Caenorhabditis elegans*, the most studied model in aging research, DAF-2 pathway and in particular DAF-16 gene, appear to be fundamental factors for its longevity as well as for its innate immunity ***(57)***. In mammalians, FOXO signaling (DAF-16 homolog) shows similar functionality and has been linked to IS homeostasis and inhibition of NF-κB activation ***(54)***. Observations of the SIRT1 activity of inhibiting NF-κB signaling and inducing FOXO signaling (that in turn potentiate NF-κB inhibition), provide a basis for the NF-κB-driven inflammaging theory ***(54)***.

Klotho mice are models used to examine senescence and accelerated aging. Non-functional mutation of Klotho gene leads to a syndrome resembling mouse aging, including osteoporosis and shortened lifespan, among others ***(54)***, while overexpression of a functional Klotho gene can extend the longevity of the animals ***(58)***, and hence it is considered an aging suppressor gene. Even if the mechanisms of Klotho gene action are not yet fully understood, it seems that the phenotype of Klotho deficient mutant mouse includes hypervitaminosis D, that induces calcium resorption from bone, an activity mediated by RANK (receptor activator of NF-κB)/RANK Ligand system of osteoclasts. Considering that osteoclast activation is controlled by the immune system, in particular by T cells which secrete RANK Ligand to activate NF-κB system, it appears that the activation of NF-κB system regulates the osteoporosis, a prominent aging phenotype, in Klotho deficient mutants ***(54)***.

## 11.6 Conflicting or Unavailable Results on Longevity in Different Species

In some cases, results obtained in animal models have not been reproduced in humans as described below for a few genes or pathways.

### *11.6.1 p66Shc*

Knocking out p66Shc in mice leads to an increase in life span ***(59)***. These results led to the hypothesis that centenarians should hypoexpress this gene ***(60)***. In contrast, we observed that dermal fibroblasts from centenarians have higher levels of p66Shc mRNA and protein than do young and middle-aged subjects ***(61)***. Thus, further studies are necessary to elucidate these discordant results.

### *11.6.2 PON1*

Recent studies in humans demonstrated that the paraoxonase 1 (*PON1*) gene seems to be associated with longevity. In a study of Italian centenarians and Irish octogenarians and nonagenarians, an association was found between the 192R allele and longevity. 192 RR genotype further enhances the survival advantage. On one hand, this finding is of interest because the 192R allele has previously been associated with increased risk of coronary heart disease. On other hand, the 192R allele shows higher enzymatic activity, and we hypothesized that its role in the metabolism of potentially toxic chemicals or other metabolic pathways may be important in survival to very old age ***(62)***. Indeed, PON1 has been widely investigated, especially for its involvement in atherosclerosis and age-related diseases. A recent review summarizes data on the role played by PON1 in aging and its possible involvement in human longevity. It focuses on the relationship between genetic polymorphisms and enzyme activity and on the ability of PON1 to counteract oxidative stress, showing the central role of the R allele and the high enzymatic PON1 activity, which seem to favor human longevity ***(63)***. The impact of the Q192R codon on the probability of attaining longevity has been clarified by a meta-analysis of the 11 studies performed between 2002 and 2008 ***(64)***.

### *11.6.3 Caloric Restriction*

Studies of the effect of CR on life spans of animals and humans have also yielded discordant results ***(65, 66)***. One explanation is the enormous flexibility of humans to adapt to new living conditions. Several studies indicate that food restriction appears to slow the aging process in rodents, mice, and other animal species.

Different authors ***(67–70)*** found that aged CR animals had better preserved physical activity. Other studies reported that a restricted food intake diet correlates positively with life span extension not only in rodents but also in other animal species, including fruit flies ***(71)***, nematodes ***(72)***, water fleas, spiders, and fish ***(68)***. Budding yeast seems to age more slowly when nutrient supply is restricted ***(73)***. What happens to the rate of aging of primates and humans when they are under food restriction condition is still unclear. Recent studies on nonhuman primates have reported changes in physiological profiles similar to those seen in rodents ***(74, 75)***, but further evidence is needed. In another study ***(76)***, CR is used to reveal divergences of aging rates in humans compared with animals. The authors suggest that these differences reside in the stability of the metabolic network, which is the capacity of the metabolic network to control and maintain an adequate redox balance in presence of random perturbations in the reaction rates of the major enzymatic processes. Long-lived species, such as humans, are characterized by highly stable networks – metabolic systems that have a strong capacity for homeostatic regulation. Short-lived species, such as mice, are characterized by weakly stable networks – with a scarce capacity to maintain their homeostatic conditions. Theoretical studies performed by Demetrius reveal that CR increases longevity by increasing the metabolic stability of the regulatory networks ***(66)***. In the case of humans, a species close to the condition of maximal metabolic stability, theoretical studies predict that CR will have a negligible effect on stability and hence no effect on maximum life span. CR may, however, have an effect on mean life span. CR may influence mean life span simply by reducing the incidence of diseases such as diabetes, atherosclerosis, and hypertension (an increase in life span of only about 3–5 years, a moderate effect) in nonobese populations ***(66)***.

Recent data indicate that life extending effects of CR in mammalians are mainly due to *SIRT1* activation ***(77, 78)***. *SIRT1* activation induced by CR inhibits NF-κB signalling pathway, and since NF-κB plays a central role in inflammation, these effects would also explain the resistance to inflammation observed in CR animals ***(79, 80)***. The link between *SIRT1* and NF-κB explains also the protective effects of CR towards metabolic syndrome in which inflammation is a crucial pathogenic mechanism ***(81)***.

We can conclude that results obtained in animal models are often not sufficiently immediately transferred to humans and thus they can not be considered totally adequate for the study of human longevity ***(16, 82)***, even if their usefulness in achieving general knowledge at different levels of many biological process (molecular, cellular, physiological, behavioral) is unquestionable.

## 11.7 Conclusions

Human aging is a much more complex phenomenon than expected. The possibility of disentangling the molecular basis of such a process can be implemented by an evolutionary and comparative approach, thus adopting and comparing many animal models from different species and taxa.

This approach is very important. Another possibility is to study human aging in the closest animal model, i.e., the nonhuman primate. Data published some years ago indicate that nonhuman primates, such as baboons, have a high degree of genetic, anatomic, and physiologic similarity with humans. Therefore, they may assist in the detection, characterization, and identification of genetic and environmental influences on human aging. Authors demonstrated the effects of genes on variations in life spans, concluding that baboon life span is under partial genetic control ***(83)***. Other authors indicated both striking similarities and differences in human mortality patterns. Female baboons (*Papio hamadryas*) share a demographic feature with aging humans, i.e., each taxon population varies primarily at the level of the Gompertz mortality intercept (frailty) and minimally in the demographic rate of aging ***(84)***. Other authors showed that chimpanzees are among the primates most likely to demonstrate prosocial behaviors, which would be of interest for possible evaluations of and effects on life span and aging ***(85)***.

In recent studies of proteasome composition and activity in the brain of *Macaca fascicularis*, we found that *M. fascicularis* primates, compared with humans, may have a different age-dependent regulation of the ubiquitin-proteasome system in specific area of the brain susceptible to age-related oxidative stress ***(86)***.

In conclusion, it seems that ad hoc models together with new in silico and high throughput strategies are urgently needed in order to further clarify human aging and longevity. These studies will accelerate identification of new immunological, metabolic, and genetic determinants of healthy aging and longevity ***(20)***.

**Acknowledgments** This work was supported by EU (European Union) Grant "PROTEOMAGE" Contract n. FP6–518230; the PRRIITT program of the Emilia-Romagna Region (and Fondi Strutturali Obiettivo 2); Italian Ministry of Health Grant "Progetto Finalizzato Studio delle differenze uomo-donna nei meccanismi patogenetici delle malattie cardiovascolari" to CF; Italian Ministry of University and Research (MiUR) PRIN 2006 Project to CF and DM (# 2006061707), SS (# 2006063387); University of Bologna Grant "Ricerca Fondamentale Orientata (RFO ex 60%) 2007" to CF, SS and MC; Roberto and Cornelia Pallotti Legacy for Cancer Research Grants to CF, SS and MC. University of Bologna Progetti Strategici 2006 grant "p53 e patologie non neoplastiche nell'anziano: uno studio multidisciplinare sul ruolo del polimorfismo al codone 72 del gene TP53" to SS.

## References

1. Franceschi C, Monti D, Sansoni P, Cossarizza A. The immunology of exceptional individuals: The lesson of centenarians. Immunol Today 1995;16:12–6.
2. Franceschi C, Monti D, Barbieri D, et al. Immunosenescence in humans: deterioration or remodelling? Int Rev Immunol 1995;12:57–74.
3. Hasty P, Campisi J, Hoeijmakers J, Van Steeg H, Vijg J. Aging and genome maintenance: Lessons from the mouse? Science 2003;299:1355–9.
4. Salmon AB, Akha AA, Buffenstein R, Miller RA. Fibroblasts from naked mole-rats are resistant to multiple forms of cell injury, but sensitive to peroxide, ultraviolet light, and endoplasmic reticulum stress. J Gerontol A Biol Sci Med Sci 2008;63:232–41.
5. Hyun M, Lee J, Lee K, May A, Bohr VA, Ahn B. Longevity and resistance to stress correlate with DNA repair capacity in Caenorhabditis elegans. Nucleic Acids Res 2008;36:1380–9.

6. Chen JB, Sun J, Jazwinski SM. Prolongation of the yeast life span by the v-Ha-RAS oncogene. Mol Microbiol 1990;4:2081–6.
7. Orr WC, Sohal RS. Effects of Cu-Zn superoxide dismutase overexpression of life span and resistance to oxidative stress in transgenic Drosophila melanogaster. Arch Biochem Biophys 1993;301:34–40.
8. Davis T, Kipling D. Telomeres and telomerase biology in vertebrates: progress towards a non-human model for replicative senescence and aging. Biogerontology 2005;6:371–85.
9. Kapahi P, Boulton ME, Kirkwood TB. Positive correlation between mammalian life span and cellular resistance to stress. Free Radic Biol Med 1999;26:495–500.
10. Kirkwood TL, Kapahi P, Shanley DP. Evolution, stress, and longevity. J Anat 2000;197 (Pt 4):587–90.
11. Holmes DJ, Ottinger MA. Birds as long-lived animal models for the study of aging. Exp Gerontol 2003;38:1365–75.
12. Martin GM, Bergman A, Barzilai N. Genetic determinants of human health span and life span: Progress and new opportunities. PLoS Genet 2007;3:e125.
13. Pollard KS, Salama SR, Lambert N, et al. An RNA gene expressed during cortical development evolved rapidly in humans. Nature 2006;443:167–72.
14. Pollard KS, Salama SR, King B, et al. Forces shaping the fastest evolving regions in the human genome. PLoS Genet 2006;2:e168.
15. Jeune B, Skytthe A, Cournil A. Handgrip strength among nonagenarians and centenarians in three European regions. J Gerontol A Biol Sci Med Sci 2006;61:707–12.
16. De Benedictis G, Franceschi C. The unusual genetics of human longevity. Sci Aging Knowledge Environ. 2006;2006:pe20.
17. Martin GM. Constitutional genetic markers of aging. Exp Gerontol 1988;23:257–70.
18. Martin GM, Austad SN, Johnson TE. Genetic analysis of aging: Role of oxidative damage and environmental stresses. Nat Genet 1996;13:25–34.
19. Partridge L, Gems D. Mechanisms of aging: Public or private? Nat Rev Genet 2002;3:165–75.
20. Franceschi C, Capri M, Monti D, et al. Inflammaging and anti-inflammaging: a systemic perspective on aging and longevity emerged from studies in humans. Mech Ageing Dev 2007;128:92–105.
21. Barker DJ. The developmental origins of chronic adult disease. Acta Paediatr Suppl 2004;93:26–33.
22. Reyes L, Mañalich R. Long-term consequences of low birth weight. Kidney Int Suppl 2005;97:S107–11.
23. Elovitz MA, Mrinalini C, Sammel MD. Elucidating the early signal transduction pathways leading to fetal brain injury in preterm birth. Pediatr Res 2006;59:50–5.
24. De Magalhaes JP. Open-minded scepticism: inferring the causal mechanisms of human aging from genetic perturbations. Ageing Res Rev 2005;4:1–22.
25. Williams GC, Knipp GT, Sinko PJ. The effect of cell culture conditions on saquinavir transport through, and interactions with, MDCKII cells overexpressing hMDR1. J Pharm Sci 2003;92:1957–67.
26. Hawkes K. Grandmothers and the evolution of human longevity. Am J Hum Biol 2003;15:380–400.
27. Kim S, Benguria A, Lai CY, Jazwinski SM. Modulation of life-span by histone deacetylase genes in Saccharomyces cerevisiae. Mol Biol Cell 1999;10:3125–36.
28. Tissenbaum HA, Guarente L. Increased dosage of a sir-2 gene extends lifespan in Caenorhabditis elegans. Nature 20018;410:227–30.
29. Rose G, Dato S, Altomare K, et al. Variability of the SIRT3 gene, human silent information regulator Sir2 homologue, and survivorship in the elderly. Exp Gerontol 2003;38:1065–70.
30. Bellizzi D, Rose G, Cavalcante P, et al. A novel VNTR enhancer within the SIRT3 gene, a human homologue of SIR2, is associated with survival at oldest ages. Genomics 2005;85:258–63.

31. Longo VD, Finch CE. Evolutionary medicine: from dwarf model systems to healthy centenarians? Science 2003;299:1342–6.
32. Kenyon C. A conserved regulatory system for aging. Cell 2001;105:165–8.
33. Hsieh CC, DeFord JH, Flurkey K, Harrison DE, Papaconstantinou J. Effects of the Pit1 mutation on the insulin signaling pathway: Implications on the longevity of the longlived Snell dwarf mouse. Mech Ageing Dev 2002;123:1245–55.
34. Dozmorov I, Bartke A, Miller RA. Array-based expression analysis of mouse liver genes: Effect of age and of the longevity mutant Prop1df. J Gerontol A Biol Sci Med Sci 2001;56:B72–80.
35. Bonafè M, Barbieri M, Marchegiani F, et al. Polymorphic variants of insulin-like growth factor I (IGF-I) receptor and phosphoinositide 3-kinase genes affect IGF-I plasma levels and human longevity: cues for an evolutionarily conserved mechanism of life span control. J Clin Endocrinol Metab 2003;88:3299–304.
36. Franceschi C, Olivieri F, Marchegiani F, et al. Genes involved in immune response/inflammation, IGF-I/insulin pathway and response to oxidative stress play a major role in the genetics of human longevity: the lesson of centenarians. Mech Ageing Dev 2005;126:351–61.
37. Van Heemst D, Beekman M, Mooijaart SP, et al. Reduced insulin/IGF-I signalling and human longevity. Aging Cell 2005;4:79–85.
38. Donehower LA, Harvey M, Slagle BL, et al. Mice deficient for p53 are developmentally normal but susceptible to spontaneous tumours. Nature 199219;356:215–21.
39. Tyner SD, Venkatachalam S, Choi J, et al. p53 mutant mice that display early ageing-associated phenotypes. Nature 20023;415:45–53.
40. García-Cao I, García-Cao M, Martín-Caballero J, et al. 'Super p53' mice exhibit enhanced DNA damage response, are tumor resistant and age normally. EMBO J 2002;21:6225–35.
41. Ko LJ, Prives C. p53: Puzzle and paradigm. Genes Dev 1996;10:1054–72.
42. Bonafe M, Salvioli S, Barbi C, et al. The different apoptotic potential of the p53 codon 72 alleles increases with age and modulates in vivo ischaemia-induced cell death. Cell Death Differ 2004;11:962–73.
43. Sullivan A, Syed N, Gasco M, et al. Polymorphism in wild-type p53 modulates response to chemotherapy in vitro and in vivo. Oncogene 2004;23:3328–37.
44. Salvioli S, Bonafé M, Barbi C, et al. p53 codon 72 alleles influence the response to anticancer drugs in cells from aged people by regulating the cell cycle inhibitor p21WAF1. Cell Cycle 2005;4:1264–71.
45. Den Reijer PM, Maier AB, Westendorp RG, van Heemst D. Influence of the TP53 codon 72 polymorphism on the cellular responses to X-irradiation in fibroblasts from nonagenarians. Mech Ageing Dev 2008;129:175–82.
46. Bonafè M, Barbi C, Storci G, et al. What studies on human longevity tell us about the risk for cancer in the oldest old: Data and hypotheses on the genetics and immunology of centenarians. Exp Gerontol 2002;37:1263–71.
47. Van Heemst D, Mooijaart SP, Beekman M, et al. Long Life Study Group. Variation in the human TP53 gene affects old age survival and cancer mortality. Exp Gerontol 2005;40:11–5.
48. Ørsted DD, Bojesen SE, Tybjaerg-Hansen A, Nordestgaard BG. Tumor suppressor p53 Arg72Pro polymorphism and longevity, cancer survival, and risk of cancer in the general population. J Exp Med 2007;204:1295–301.
49. Wasserman SA. Toll signaling: The enigma variations. Curr Opin Genet Dev 2000;10:497–502.
50. Hoffmann JA. The immune response of Drosophila. Nature 2003;426:33–8.
51. Waterhouse RM, Kriventseva EV, Meister S, et al. Evolutionary Dynamics of Immune-Related Genes and Pathways in Disease-Vector Mosquitoes. Science 2007;316:1738–43.
52. Wang XW, Tan NS, Ho B, Ding JL. Evidence for the ancient origin of the NF-kappaB/IkappaB cascade: its archaic role in pathogen infection and immunity. Proc Natl Acad Sci U S A 2006;103:4204–9.
53. Pujol N, Link EM, Liu LX, et al. A reverse genetic analysis of components of the Toll signaling pathway in Caenorhabditis elegans. Curr Biol 2001;11:809–21.

54. Salminen A, Huuskonen J, Ojala J, Kauppinen A, Kaarniranta K, Suuronen T. Activation of innate immunity system during aging: NF-κB signaling is the molecular culprit of inflamm-aging. Ageing Res Rev, 2008;7:83-–105.
55. Guarente L. Sir2 links chromatin silencing, metabolism, and aging. Genes Dev 2000;14:1021–6.
56. Sinclair DA. Paradigms and pitfalls of yeast longevity research. Mech Ageing Dev 2002;123:857–67.
57. Henderson ST, Bonafe M, Johnson TE. daf-16 protects the nematode *Caenorhabditis elegans* during food deprivation. J Gerontol A Biol Sci Med Sci 2006;61:444–60.
58. Kurosu H, Yamamoto M, Clark JD, et al. Suppression of aging in mice by the hormone Klotho. Science 2005;309:1829–33.
59. Migliaccio E, Giorgio M, Mele S, et al. The p66shc adaptor protein controls oxidative stress response and life span in mammals. Nature 1999;402:309–13.
60. Purdom S, Chen QM. p66(Shc): At the crossroad of oxidative stress and the genetics of aging. Trends Mol Med 2003;9:206–10.
61. Pandolfi S, Bonafè M, Di Tella L, et al. p66(shc) is highly expressed in fibroblasts from centenarians. Mech Ageing Dev 2005;126:839–44.
62. Rea IM, McKeown PP, McMaster D, et al. Paraoxonase polymorphisms PON1 192 and 55 and longevity in Italian centenarians and Irish nonagenarians. A pooled analysis. Exp Gerontol 2004;39:629–35.
63. Marchegiani F, Marra M, Olivieri F, et al. Paraoxonase 1: Genetics and activities during aging. Rejuvenation Res 2008;11:113–27.
64. Lescai L, Marchegiani F, Franceschi C. PON1 is a longevity gene: the results of a meta-analysis. Ageing Res Rev 2009; in press.
65. Shanley DR, Kirkwood TBL. Caloric restriction does not enhance longevity in all species and is unlikely to do so in humans. Biogerontology 2006;7:165–8.
66. Demetrius L. Aging in mouse and human systems: a comparative study. Ann N Y Acad Sci 2006;1067:66–82.
67. McCay C, Crowell M, Maynard L. The effect of retarded growth upon the length of the life span and upon the ultimate body size. J Nutr 1935;10:63–79.
68. Weindruch R, Walford RL. The retardation of aging and disease by dietary restriction. Springfield, IL: Charles C. Thomas Publisher Ltd, 1988.
69. Sprott RL. Diet and calorie restriction. Exp Gerontol 1997;32:205–14.
70. Means LW, Higgins JL, Fernandez TJ. Midlife onset of dietary restriction extends life and prolongs cognitive-functioning. Physiol Behav 1993;54:503–8.
71. Chapman T, Partridge L. Female fitness in Drosophila melanogaster: an interaction between the effect of nutrition and of encounter rate with males. Proc R Soc Lond B Biol Sci 1996;263:755–9.
72. Houthoofd K, Braeckman BP, Lenaerts I, et al. Axenic growth up-regulates mass specific metabolic rate, stress resistance, and extends life span in Caenorhabditis elegans. Exp Gerontol 2002;37:1371–8.
73. Jiang JC, Jaruga E, Repnevskaya MV, Jazwinski SM. An intervention resembling caloric restriction prolongs life span and retards aging in yeast. FASEB J 2000;14:2135–7.
74. Ramsey JJ, Colman RJ, Binkley NC, et al. Dietary restriction and aging in rhesus monkeys: The University of Wisconsin study. Exp Gerontol 2000;35:1131–49.
75. Lane MA, Mattison JA, Roth GS, Brant LJ, Ingram DK. Effects of long-term diet restriction on aging and longevity in primates remain uncertain. J Gerontol Ser A Biol Sci Med Sci 2004;59:405–7.
76. Demetrius L. Caloric restriction, metabolic rate, and entropy. J Gerontol Ser A Biol Sci Med Sci 2004;59:B902–15.
77. Le Bourg E, Rattan SI. Can dietary restriction increase longevity in all species, particularly in human beings? Introduction to a debate among experts. Biogerontology 2006;7:123–5.
78. Chen D, Guarente L. SIR2: A potential target for calorie restriction mimetics. Trends Mol Med 2007;13:64–71.
79. Holloszy JO, Fontana L. Caloric restriction in humans. Exp Gerontol 2007;42:709–12.

80. Morgan TE, Wong AM, Finch CE. Anti-inflammatory mechanisms of dietary restriction in slowing aging processes. Interdiscip Top Gerontol 2007;35:83–97.
81. Guarente L. Sirtuins as potential targets for metabolic syndrome. Nature 2006;444:868–74.
82. Capri M, Monti D, Salvioli S, et al. Complexity of anti-immunosenescence strategies in humans. Artif Organs 2006;30:730–42.
83. Martin LJ, Mahaney MC, Bronikowski AM, Dee Carey K, Dyke B, Comuzzie AG. Lifespan in captive baboons is heritable. Mech Ageing Dev 2002;123:1461–7.
84. Bronikowski AM, Alberts SC, Altmann J, Packer C, Carey KD, Tatar M. The aging baboon: Comparative demography in a non-human primate. Proc Natl Acad Sci U S A 2002;99:9591–5.
85. Silk JB, Brosnan SF, Vonk J, et al. Chimpanzees are indifferent to the welfare of unrelated group members. Nature 2005;437:1357–9.
86. Bellavista E, Mishto M, Santoro A, Bertoni-Freddari C, Sessions RB, Franceschi C. Immunoproteasome in Macaca fascicularis: No age-dependent modification of abundance and activity in the brain and insight into an in silico structural model. Rejuvenation Res 2008;11:73–82.

# Index